C000265493

Raw Food Cookbook and Diet

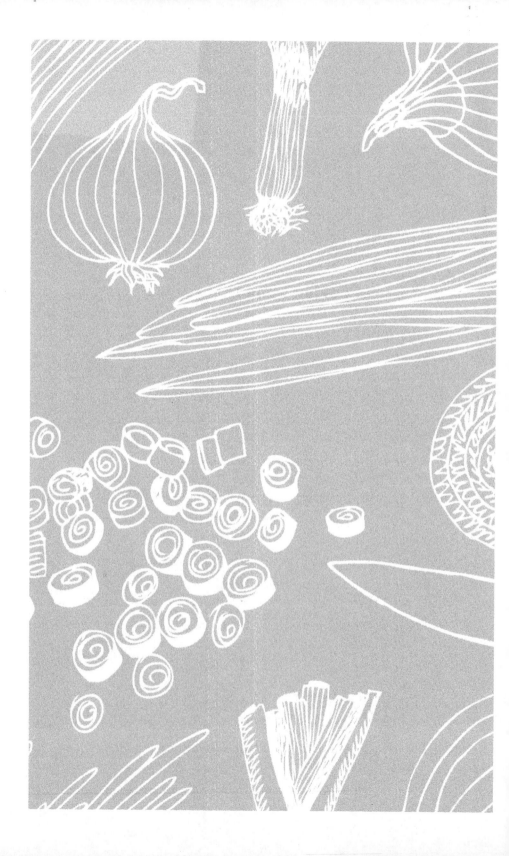

Raw Food Cookbook and Diet

75 EASY, DELICIOUS, AND FLEXIBLE
RECIPES FOR A RAW FOOD DIET

ROCKRIDGE
PRESS

Contents

CHAPTER EIGHT

Soups

CHAPTER NINE

Salads

CHAPTER THIRTEEN

Snacks and Kid-Friendly Recipes

Introduction

The idea of a raw food diet appears to be quite simple: between 75 and 100 percent of one's diet should be composed of raw or living foods. This certainly sounds like an easy diet to follow. How hard could it be to prepare raw ingredients? Simply wash and serve, right? But it's actually a little more complicated than that to do it right and ensure that you follow a healthful diet.

Once you make the decision to eat raw, you don't need to turn off your stove and swear off cheesecake. First, it's never a good idea to jump into a new diet without a transition period, especially a raw diet. The take-no-prisoners approach can cause unpleasant serious detox symptoms as your body gets used to the new diet. But as you make the transition, you'll be pleasantly surprised to find that many of your familiar favorite ingredients have different textures when not heated. Cooking completely changes the taste and mouthfeel of food products. If you want to reap the full health benefits of the raw food diet, it is best to work up to about 75 percent raw foods.

It might seem difficult to transition into this diet if you have a health condition you are trying to improve. Be patient. Even just a few raw food meals will quickly raise your energy levels. Before long, your hair will shine and your skin will be almost luminous.

There's a good chance you will lose weight as well. It's logical to assume that weight loss will occur with a diet of predominantly fresh fruits, vegetables, and lean protein that is low in fat and high in fiber and water content. So if your health and well-being are important to you, the raw food diet might be the answer.

CHAPTER ONE

What Is Raw Food?

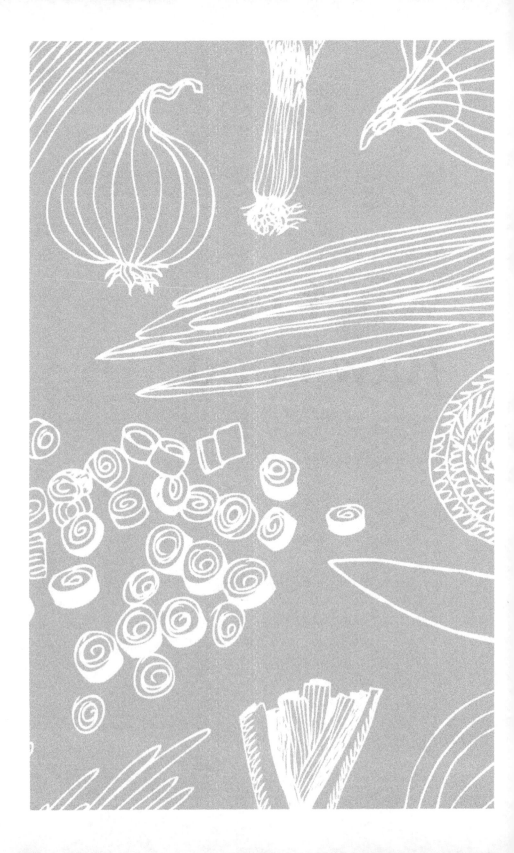

What Is Raw Food?

The basic raw food diet focuses on not cooking food above 118 degrees F. It contains fruits, vegetables, sprouted seeds, soaked grains, dried fruit, miso, nut-based cheeses, rolled grains, nuts, and seeds. This diet is quite close to what most health professionals advocate for a healthful eating plan. Unfortunately, the preparation and planning of these products can be a little more time-consuming and expensive than standard processed convenience foods. These drawbacks can end up scaring people away from even trying this lifestyle choice.

Eating raw or living food is not a new concept. Human beings have consumed food in this state for most of the history of our race. Cooking food products is a relatively new step in the path from field to fork. It's interesting to note that many serious health concerns such as obesity and heart disease have worsened since processed cooked foods became the norm.

THE HISTORY OF RAW FOOD

Homo sapiens, who started cooking their food after the discovery of fire, are the only species to consume cooked foods. Some anthropologists, such as Dr. Richard Wrangham, claim we owe our large brain, body physique, jaw shape, and teeth configuration to this switch. While the debate continues on that theory, it is undisputed that the human diet was raw for tens or hundreds of thousands of years.

Raw food diets are well documented throughout history, with many cultures such as India and Iran following a largely raw vegan diet. The evolution of an actual raw diet plan for health and well-being really started in the last few centuries with several pioneers and researchers.

- **c. 460–370 BC:** Hippocrates, the Father of Medicine, and Pythagoras, noted Greek philosopher and mathematician, were credited with eating a largely raw vegan diet. This is speculation, however, since what people consumed that far back in history is largely unknown.

- **1850:** Sylvester Graham, a Presbyterian minister, started the American Vegetarian Society and was instrumental in promoting the vegan, mostly raw movement. His focus was not only health-based in the sense that we understand it now; he believed that the consumption of animal-based by-products aroused lust, which he wished to eradicate.

- **Between 1890 and 1922:** Arnold Ehret, a health educator, cured himself of Bright's disease by fasting and following a predominantly raw vegetarian diet. His clinics in Switzerland and California used these techniques as a basis for their healing therapies.

- **Between 1895 and 1900:** Dr. Max Otto Bircher-Benner, creator of muesli, conducted many experiments that investigated the power of raw foods to heal. He even cured himself of jaundice using a vegan, mostly raw diet. The results of his research led to the opening of the Bircher-Benner Clinic in Zurich, Switzerland, which is known for healing many people considered to have incurable diseases. Bircher-Benner taught that food was not simply a means to satiate; it should keep the body strong and vibrant as well.

- **The early 1900s:** Dr. Max Gerson pioneered a healing technique for cancer that focused on diet, specifically raw foods and a great deal of water. The conclusions reached in his study "The Cure of Advanced Cancer by Diet Therapy: A Summary of 30 Years of Clinical Experimentation" are still used today to treat diabetes, heart disease, and cancer.

- **The 1930s:** Dr. Paul Kouchakoff conducted research that studied the body's reaction in response to dangerous pathogens. This reaction, called digestive leukocytosis, is produced when cooked foods are eaten but not when raw foods are consumed.

- **1933:** Noted scientist E. B. Forbes linked cooked foods to dental degeneration. Cooked foods are more prone to stick to the teeth and create a favorable environment for acid fermentation.

- **1936:** Weston A. Price, a dentist, also blamed cooked foods for dental issues, observing that the consumption of processed foods had overtaken nutrient-rich ones and that the trend of tooth decay could be linked to that switch.

- **Between 1941 and 1981:** Dr. Edward Howell, a physician, wrote three books that claimed the body has to work harder to process cooked foods.

He also advanced the popular raw food theory that food enzymes play an important role in digesting food.

- **The 1960s:** Viktoras Kulvinskas and Ann Wigmore founded the Hippocrates Institute, which is devoted to the practice of eating raw foods for health and spiritual wellness. This institute continues its work today.
- **The 1970s and 1980s:** The raw food movement started to make its way into the mainstream population. Books such as *Survival into the 21st Century* by Viktoras Kulvinskas and *The New Raw Energy* by Leslie Kenton inspired interest in this type of diet. Several raw food chefs introduced delicious raw meals that further peaked interest. Many well-known celebrities joined the raw food movement, creating buzz in the media, and soon raw food was touted as the magical solution to increased health, beauty, and youthfulness.

DO ANY CULTURES EAT ONLY RAW FOOD?

Raw food diets have appeared throughout history in many different cultures. No single culture stands out as consuming only raw foods, although some are known to follow a partial raw food lifestyle, most often out of necessity or lack of means to cook rather than for health benefits.

One group of people linked to raw food is the Hunza, who live in a remote region in Pakistan. These long-living people apparently do not exhibit many of the diseases found in more industrialized societies. Researchers theorize that the Hunzas' largely raw diet is a major contributor to their good health. While these claims of longevity may be true, the lack of birth records and other records make it very difficult to verify. Another culture with similar claims and similar issues relating to absent statistics is the Okinawans of Japan.

One of the few documented examples of a culture that ate a majority of raw food is the Eskimo. The word *Eskimo* literally means "one who eats raw." When looking at this group, some revealing health statistics become apparent. Eskimo people who still follow their traditional diet present no arteriosclerosis, high blood pressure, obesity, stroke, or heart disease. These Eskimos also rarely suffer from minor ailments such as digestive problems, sinus issues, headaches, or fatigue.

IS THERE ONLY ONE WAY TO GO RAW?

The raw food diet offers many different variations, depending on the ideology of the person embarking on this lifestyle choice. In its purest form, the raw food diet is quite simply to eat only raw foods. This can be a very challenging, strict way of eating, one that requires a great deal of conviction and self-control. Even among those people who eat 100 percent raw foods, there are different opinions on what can or cannot be included, such as maple syrup or unpasteurized dairy products. These decisions are entirely your choice, and there is no one right approach beyond doing what works for you, your daily routine, and your health. The most common variations of this diet usually recommend eating at least 75 percent raw, unless you are transitioning to raw eating. Some different approaches to the raw food diet include:

In Transition

After some research, you've decided to try a raw food diet. Basically, you want to get your toes wet without making a full-splash commitment, so you start adding raw foods to your daily routine. This could mean a green smoothie for breakfast or a hearty salad for dinner with plenty of vegetables snacks throughout the day. The goal is to slowly work up to whatever percentage of raw foods you are comfortable with. Some people stay in this eating pattern indefinitely.

Strict Raw Vegan

The raw diet is actually a relatively easy transition for practicing vegans since many of the ingredients are the same; you just have to give up the cooking of your food. Raw vegan is similar to regular vegan in that you restrict the consumption of all animal products and concentrate solely on fruit, vegetables, nuts, seeds, and sprouted products. Within this group exist several more specialized subgroups that practice even stricter eating plans. These include people who eat only fruit (fruitarians), those who eat only sprouted seeds (sproutarians), and those who consume only raw juices (juicearians).

Raw Vegetarian

Similar to raw vegan, this group also includes some dairy products and raw honey in their diet. Because dairy products need to be raw or unpasteurized to meet the raw food requirements, it's important to find reputable suppliers to ensure food safety.

Flexible Raw Omnivore

This is the most flexible raw food diet variation and the easiest to follow. Basically, you can eat whatever you wish (with an eye on staying healthy) as long as you consume at least 75 percent raw products. Some raw food purists would not call this a raw diet, but as long as processed foods are not on the menu, this choice is fine. This restriction includes "processed" beef or chicken from farms that use hormones, antibiotics, and genetically enhanced feed.

Raw Food Animal Diets

Two diets include the eating of raw animal products, the raw Paleolithic diet and the primal diet. The former avoids the same items found on the cooked diet, such as dairy, legumes, and grains, and focuses on raw meats, raw fish, raw eggs, and some raw vegetables. The primal diet is made up of raw meats, raw organ meats, raw honey, raw dairy, and some vegetable and fruit juices.

The variety of the listed approaches allow you to tailor a raw food plan to your needs. This greatly increases your chances of sticking to your new diet.

CHAPTER TWO

Cooked versus Raw Food

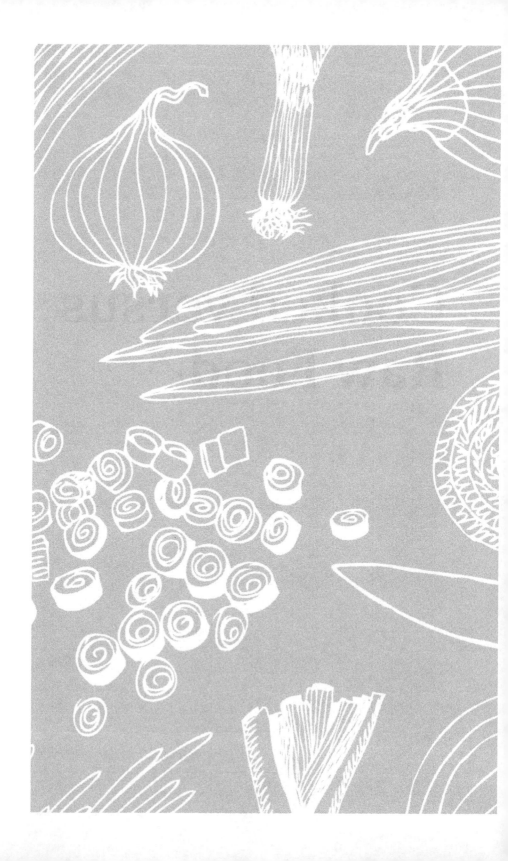

Cooked versus Raw Food

Since the foundation of the raw diet concerns the benefits of eating raw products rather than cooked, it's important to understand what happens when you place that steak on a grill or blanch your vegetables. Cooking is an intensely personal experience and can evoke many memories and traditions, and eliminating this can be difficult. The trick to transitioning to a raw diet is understanding that you will still be creating delicious dishes that you and your family will enjoy.

WHAT OCCURS WHEN FOOD IS COOKED?

Cooking is a process that involves breaking down (processing) foods and heating them up. This process causes chemical and physical changes to occur. The question might be why would we do this to products we intend to eat?

Safety

People often cook their food because eating it raw can cause sickness. The most common foods that might cause food poisoning are meats, seafood, and dairy products. Bacteria thrive and grow between 41 and 140 degrees F, which means to kill them you need to heat your foods higher. Food poisoning can also occur on produce that has not been washed thoroughly. Unhygienic growing, picking, and handling of fruits and vegetables is the most common cause of this contamination.

Flavor and Color

Even though raw foods in their natural state are delicious in their simplicity and pure flavor, cooking can make food taste and look better. Several different processes create these alterations in your food.

1. **Caramelization.** This process produces a chain reaction of chemical changes, mostly in high-carbohydrate foods, that in the end produce a color and flavor modification. In essence, the sugar in food melts and boils as heat is applied and breaks down into smaller molecules, such as fructose and glucose. These molecules undergo even more intricate chemical reactions, producing hundreds of different flavor compounds. The exact compounds depend on what food is being heated. During caramelization the caramel molecules are produced, which create the appetizing brown color you see in many cooked dishes.

2. **Loss of color.** Have you ever noticed that blanching green beans causes a series of color changes? This happens because heat creates changes depending on the length of heat application. When heat is applied to the green beans, oxygen leaves the pigment, creating a bright attractive green color. If you continue to apply heat, however, it causes the green beans to release acids, which in turn convert the chlorophyll into grayish or dark green pigments called pheophyll and pheophytin b. Cooking can affect the pigments in many other fruits and vegetables, primarily because these are the foods that contain the most pigments.

3. **The Maillard reaction.** When food is heated, a reaction occurs between the sugars (glucose, lactose, and fructose) and an amino acid that sets off cascading changes, which creates color and flavor alterations in the food.

4. **Starch degradation.** All tubers and seeds contain a polysaccharide starch, which is basically glucose units strung together with glycosidic bonds. These bonds break when heat is applied to the food, causing the glucose molecules to be released. This process produces a pleasing sweetness in cooked foods.

Vitamins

A main reason many people prefer eating raw foods is because they believe cooking leaches the vitamins and other nutrients out of the products. Vitamins are essential to good health and can be either water- or fat-soluble. Water-soluble vitamins are found in fruits and vegetables, which have a high water content, while fat-soluble vitamins are often found in dairy products, oils, and fish. Fat- and water-soluble vitamins are impacted greatly by cooking methods that involve either fat or water. For example, placing vegetables in boiling water can leach the vitamins out of the food. The extent of vitamin loss is also affected by the length of time the food is exposed to heat. Quick-cooking methods such as stir-frying create much less loss than roasting or braising.

Texture

An important aspect of any dish, texture is strongly influenced by cooking.

- **Polysaccharide degradation.** When you apply heat to vegetables and other plant products, they become soft. Why? During the cooking process the polysaccharides that provide structure and crispness (pectin and cellulose) are broken down into smaller molecules, creating softness and, in extreme cases, mushiness.
- **Polysaccharide gelatinization.** One of the quickest ways to create a thick gravy or custard is through the use of products such as cornstarch. Cornstarch contains a polysaccharide starch made up of two components, amylose and amylopectin. When you heat cornstarch in water (or another liquid), the starch swells and the amylose leaks out to create a lattice structure, which traps the water molecules. This creates the thickening in sauces.
- **Protein denaturation.** Proteins, found in food products such as eggs, vegetables, nuts, and legumes, contain amino acids, which are linked by peptic bonds in different configurations. The different amino acids are held together by hydrogen bonds to create three-dimensional protein molecules. When proteins are cooked, they vibrate, which can break the hydrogen bonds and cause the protein to fall apart into separate amino acids. These acids rearrange, which changes the texture of the food substantially. For example, egg white becomes firm when cooked.

Cooking Creates Beneficial Molecules

Cooking certain foods creates molecules that make antioxidants more readily available to the body. For example, studies have shown that anticancer compounds such as lycopene are absorbed more easily by the human body when vegetables are cooked. This might be due to the destruction of the connective bands of the cell matrix during the cooking process.

IS THERE A CONNECTION BETWEEN COOKED FOOD AND CANCER?

Although cooking can create changes in food that are favorable, it can also generate undesirable compounds such as carcinogens. Carcinogens are cancer-causing agents, which are a serious health threat. Certain cooking processes create more carcinogens than others. Curing meat with sodium nitrate can cause carcinogen compounds called nitrosamines, which are also found in tobacco and produced in fried or smoked foods. Countless studies detail the dangers of barbecuing food, because charring creates carcinogens called heterocyclic amines.

The link between cooked foods and cancer is not just found in meats. Recent studies have found that cooking carbohydrates and other foods at high temperatures can produce a cancer-causing chemical called acrylamide. This odorless white chemical, used to treat sewage and manufacture dyes and plastics, is found in potato chips, rice, cereal, French fries, and even bread. Any food that is fried, baked, grilled, or roasted could contain this chemical, with high-carbohydrate foods being particularly susceptible. Because researchers cannot pinpoint exactly what part of the cooking process creates this chemical, it is difficult to eliminate it.

Another interesting theory concerns the discovery made in the 1900s that pancreatic enzymes can digest cancer cells. Enzyme therapy has been used with great success in Europe and parts of the United States to cure or control cancer. Cooking foods is thought by raw food enthusiasts to deplete the amount of natural enzymes found in the food, which in turn can create a low level of enzymes in the body. This means the body is unable to fight off cancer cells as they form.

WHY ARE ENZYMES IMPORTANT IN THE RAW FOOD DIET?

Enzymes, proteins that exist to catalyze the chemical reactions throughout the body's systems, are crucial to the body and affect every part of it. All the cells in the body produce enzymes for their own specific activities, such as digestive enzymes produced by glands in the digestive tract.

The raw food diet focuses on the idea that cooking food above 118 degrees F destroys the naturally occurring enzymes in the food. Followers of this diet also believe that all natural food ingredients contain the enzymes required to efficiently digest that food. When those naturally occurring enzymes are destroyed by cooking, the body must do all the work. The theory states the body cannot produce the exact combination of enzymes needed by the food consumed to effectively digest it, which leads to incomplete digestion and blocked body systems. This breakdown in the system means the pancreas has to do extra work, creating more enzymes to try to break down the food effectively. After years of overwork, the pancreas cannot produce enough enzymes, which can result in low enzyme levels in the body and other health issues.

Another theory to consider is that some scientists and nutritionists believe there is a finite amount of enzymes available in the body for our lifetime. Depleting this reserve to digest cooked food has health effects later in life and can even shorten your life. Studies have revealed that an eighty-five-year-old man has approximately 33 percent of the enzyme levels of an eighteen-year-old. This deficit can affect cell division, the immune system, brain activity, and energy levels.

This raw-food-enzyme theory is subject to debate in the scientific world. Some researchers believe that when food reaches the stomach, more than 90 percent of the enzymes are destroyed anyway. Although foods do have enzyme activity, some scientists also think that this is not a replacement for digestive enzymes in the body. Enzymes in plants and other raw foods are simply digested along with all the other parts of the food. There are two sides to every theory, and supporting studies bolster both sides. Whether the raw-food-enzyme theory is correct or not, there is no argument that people are healthier when adding a large quantity of fresh vegetables and fruits to their diet.

CHAPTER THREE

Processed versus Natural

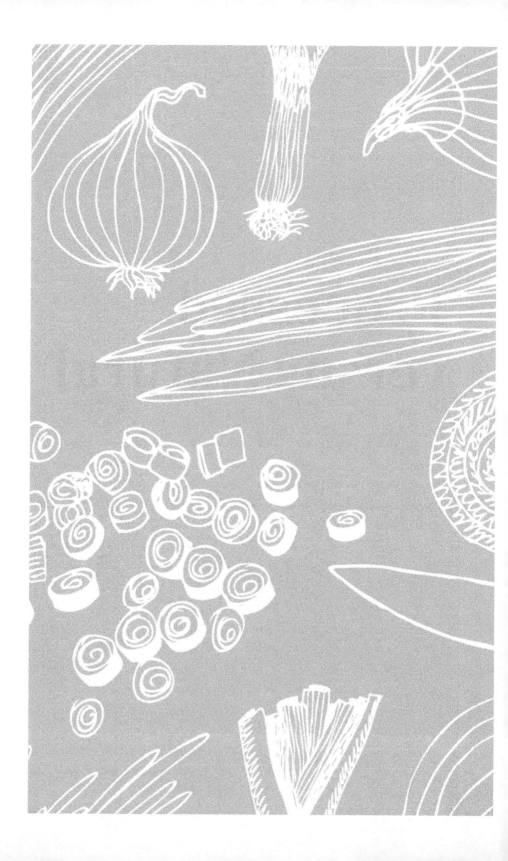

Processed versus Natural

HOW DID MODERN DIETS GO FROM WHOLE FOODS TO PROCESSED FOODS?

Food processing changes raw ingredients into other forms to increase food safety and shelf life, and to enhance taste and texture. Food processing has been around in some form or another since early man. Early processing techniques included preserving foods using salt or by sun-drying foods. Similar preservation and processing procedures are found in almost every culture, indicating that safe, available food was a concern for every human being no matter where and when. These early food-processing examples all used whole fresh foods as a starting point and did not really change the product drastically or add elements that were harmful to human beings.

Modern food processing techniques initially came about due to a military need. A sealed bottling technique was invented in 1809 by Nicolas Appert to preserve food for the French troops. This technique eventually led to canning the following year. Soon preserved food began to be mass-produced in large factories through the processes of canning, pasteurizing, sweetening, coloring, and concentrating with the goal of providing a safer, tastier product that was long-lasting, easier to transport, and above all, convenient. Two hundred years later, we ask ourselves, why we should slave over a hot stove creating meals from scratch when it is so convenient to just pop a TV dinner into the microwave? Advanced modern technologies and genetically enhanced crops make the range of processed foods available to the consumer almost endless. But with these advances in modern food processing has come a disturbing increase in obesity and other diet-related diseases. People have started to wonder whether the human body has actually benefited from all these processed foods, and some have begun to swing back in favor of a more natural diet. This burgeoning whole-food movement has been fertile ground for the development of diets such as veganism, Paleo, and the raw food diet, which feature fruits, vegetables, whole grains, and other unaltered ingredients.

ARE HUMAN BEINGS GENETICALLY PREDISPOSED TO EAT UNPROCESSED FOODS?

One theory that contributed to the development of the raw food diet is that human beings are not equipped physically to digest all the grains, dairy, legumes, and refined sugars found in processed foods. Because our digestive system has not evolved as quickly as our food preparation and preservation techniques, the modern diet has led to obesity and the plethora of serious diseases seen today. The solution is to try to eat foods that are close to what our hunter-gatherer ancestors consumed. Since we don't actually know what Stone Age humans ate with any certainty, we have to eliminate what we know they didn't eat. The rise of animal husbandry and agriculture along with industrialization added dairy, grains, legumes, and processed foods to the modern diet. When you eliminate these foods, studies have shown that cholesterol, blood pressure, blood sugar, and weight are also reduced significantly.

Does this mean we are genetically predisposed to consume more natural unprocessed foods? Dr. Loren Cordain, a leading expert in the diet practiced by our Stone Age ancestors, thought our modern processed diet was unnatural and damaging, so he developed the Paleo diet. At the root of this popular diet are lean meats, fresh fruits, plenty of vegetables, seafood, and no processed foods. The health benefits from eating a diet rich in whole nutrient-packed foods are numerous, and the risk of developing diseases such as cancer and diabetes is certainly reduced, Dr. Cordain contends. The Paleo diet is quite similar to the raw food diet in some respects, and many people make the jump from cooked Paleo to raw Paleo when they realize Stone Age humans probably didn't cook either. Whether modern humans should mimic their ancestors or not is an ongoing debate. What isn't in question is the fact that it is healthier to avoid processed foods whenever possible.

WHAT HAPPENS TO NATURAL FOODS WHEN THEY ARE PROCESSED?

In our modern world, food is processed, packaged, and placed on the shelves and dairy cases of our supermarkets. As consumers we often forget that there is a substantial amount of additives in our foods and that the food has been often altered during processing, which can remove valuable nutrients. A whole range of changes can occur during the food production process, from growing through preparation and packaging and shipping, which makes most processed foods less viable sources of healthful nutrients.

Growing and Fertilizing

One of the most common types of fertilizer used in commercial farming is nitrogen. Nitrogen can affect the amount of vitamin C found in growing fruits and vegetables. Soil contributes to the nutrient levels of the produce grown in it, but industrialized farming methods are reducing the mineral and vitamin content in the soil, most significantly, magnesium. This means even if you are eating a healthful, vegetable-packed diet, you might not be getting what you need, depending on where the produce was grown.

Milling

Another common processing method, milling affects the nutritional value of whole foods. Grains are usually milled, which means their husks are removed. The husks are packed full of phytochemicals, minerals, fiber, and B vitamins. Products produced with white flour are less healthful than their whole-grain counterparts because of the removal of these husks.

Extrusion

This is a process that is used on whole grains or a slurry of grains to produce breakfast cereal. The grains are passed through the extruder at high pressure to create the cute O's and puffed rice found on many breakfast tables. The end product is then sprayed with a light coating of sugar and oil to keep the shapes together and add texture. This process destroys almost all of the nutrients in the grains and, more disturbingly, can turn the grain proteins into neurotoxins.

Canning

Whole foods that are canned undergo an extensive processing journey that destroys many of the water-soluble vitamins (vitamin C and B vitamins) naturally found in them. The canning process involves a quick blanching (heating with steam or water) of the food to kill any existing bacteria before packing it into cans. The temperature required to eliminate microbacteria also removes some of the taste and texture of the food.

Pasteurization

Heating liquid foods such as milk and fruit juices to specific temperatures destroys microorganisms, which increases food safety. But processing milk this way also tends to turn the proteins in milk allergenic, making it hard to digest. While pasteurization can make products safer and extend their shelf life, it also can remove beneficial bacteria along with other harmful microorganisms and can affect the taste. You might not even recognize milk straight from the cow if you have been raised on store-bought products. Pasteurized juices can lose some of their vitamin C in this process as well.

Debittering

Because people like good-tasting food, the food industry routinely removes substances called phytonutrients because they are bitter and astringent. But phytonutrients are crucial for helping the body run effectively and fight chronic disease, so processing food in this manner reduces its nutritional value.

Of course not all processing methods are equally harmful to foods. Some will increase the convenience of storage or preserve the food without destroying much of its nutritional value.

Dehydration

One of the most popular processing techniques practiced by raw foodists, dehydration often turns one food into a completely different type of food. For example, juicy plump grapes become sweet, chewy raisins. Dried foods also are more energy dense than the original product. Dehydrating can take some vitamin C out of produce, but overall it is a great way to preserve and enhance food.

Freezing

Raw food enthusiasts usually allow this technique because it does not impact nutrients very much and it is a highly effective way to preserve food. If the food is just picked, it should be fine except for some flavor loss. One possible concern with freezing is that fruit can become mushy when frozen. This is fine for food destined for smoothies but not too palatable for any other type of culinary application.

Prepping

When preparing raw foods, there is often a great deal of peeling, cutting, and chopping of fresh produce. If you routinely peel your fruits and vegetables, you are removing valuable vitamins and nutrients along with the tough skin. Some skins contain a great deal of fiber and should be left on whenever possible, as long as you take the time to wash the produce well.

WHAT ROLE DO PHYTONUTRIENTS PLAY IN NUTRITION?

You might not know what a phytonutrient is, but every time you admire the deep red of a ripe tomato or inhale the heady scent of fresh garlic you are experiencing them. Phytonutrients aren't nutrients in the same class as protein or vitamins, but they are instrumental in protecting against many diseases and helping the human body stay healthy. There are tens of thousands of phytonutrients, and because they have been prevalent in health news over the last decade, at least a few names should ring a bell. Some of the most common ones are beta-carotene, flavonoids, and lutein. The health benefits of phytonutrients include:

- **Allylic sulfides.** Improves the immune system, reduces bad cholesterol, and helps protect the cells from carcinogens
- **Carotenoids.** Improves the immune system and cuts the risk of most diseases
- **Catechins.** Neutralizes free radicals and helps prevent certain types of cancer
- **Coumarins.** Helps prevent blood from clotting
- **Ellagic acid.** Helps protect against cancer
- **Flavonoids.** Prevents inflammation, enhances the effect of vitamin C, and strengthens blood vessels
- **Flavonols.** Cuts the risk of heart disease, cancers, and asthma
- **Glucosinolates.** Helps stop the growth of cancer cells
- **Limonoids.** Helps detoxify cancer-causing agents by triggering enzymes in the liver
- **Lycopene.** Helps lower the risk of prostate cancer
- **Phytoestrogens.** Helps prevent bone loss and cuts the risk of endometrial cancer in women
- **Polyphenols.** Reduces the risk of heart disease and the levels of systematic inflammation

- **Resveratrol.** Helps reduce the risk of cancer and cardiovascular disease
- **Saponins.** Helps prevent cancer cells from multiplying and lowers LDL (bad) cholesterol

HOW CAN YOU ENSURE THAT YOU ARE GETTING ENOUGH PHYTONUTRIENTS?

If you follow a well-balanced raw diet consisting of a broad array of colorful produce, you won't have to worry about whether you are consuming enough phytonutrients. The colors found in vegetables and fruit are great indicators of phytonutrients, and the deeper the hue, the more phytonutrients. Try to eat snowy cauliflower and garlic as well. They also contain these healthful compounds. Choose a variety of unblemished, vibrant-colored produce every day to ensure the phytonutrient content is high. Soil conditions, plant species, and processing techniques will all affect the amount of phytonutrients in any given fruit or vegetable, so buy organic whenever possible.

WHAT ARE THE BENEFITS OF ORGANIC FOODS?

The word *organic* is often applied to produce, meats, and grains to refer to the way these products are grown and raised. Organic food used to be found only at boutique grocery stores and farmers markets but is now prominently displayed in most supermarkets, making it more mainstream and accessible. What does that organic label stuck to your apple mean, and how is that apple different from the other conventionally farmed apple sitting next to it with a lower price?

At a minimum, organic farming refers to the growing of crops using minimal or no artificial pesticides and fertilizers. Organic farming is also practiced with an eye on water and soil conservation, while trying to minimize the environmental damage done by the chemicals and pesticides used in conventional farming. Many countries and states have stringent guidelines about what constitutes organic and when a food can be called organic; farmers cannot label their products organic without following these regulations, which sometimes require certification. Be sure to look for the organic label on items. Products touted as "natural," "hormone-free," and "free range," while probably better than conventional ones, aren't necessarily organic.

ARE ORGANIC FOODS BETTER?

Many raw foodists insist that organic is the only choice to make when following this diet, due to both health and philosophical reasons. Buying organic foods strictly for health reasons is not necessarily justified and can be completely unrealistic with respect to budget and geography for some people. Organic foods are more expensive, and often people who live in remote or colder locations can't find all the necessary types of ingredients. If you aren't eating totally organic, don't despair. Simply making the switch to mostly raw is what matters.

While organic foods have some advantages, studies have shown they are no more nutritious than conventionally produced unprocessed products, so don't buy them strictly for nutrition considerations. Some people believe organic food tastes better. This could be true because organic fruits and vegetables are not artificially ripened. A sun-ripened tomato eaten fresh off the vine is infinitely tastier than one picked green and shipped thousands of miles in a truck. Organic produce isn't coated in herbicides, pesticides, and other chemicals used to protect crops from diseases and bugs. They are also free of the preservatives, ripeners, sweeteners, and other additives used to enhance the shelf life and appearance of conventionally produced items. So if these aspects of organic foods appeal to you, then by all means search them out and buy them. But if it is not possible to eat only organic, then be sensible and don't stress. Simply wash your ingredients thoroughly, and enjoy the benefits of following a healthful raw food diet.

Balance and the Raw Food Diet

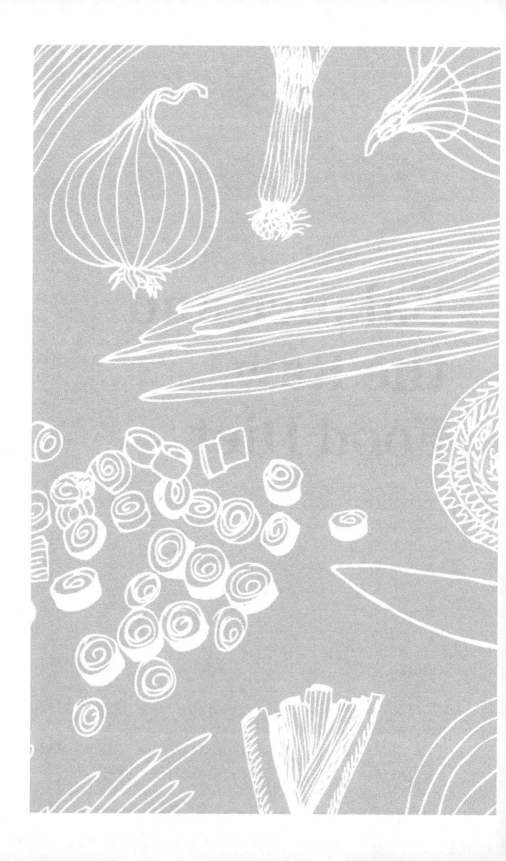

Balance and the Raw Food Diet

WHAT IS A SENSIBLE APPROACH TO THE RAW DIET?

Since every person is different and has individual health needs, diets cannot be one size fits all. The reasons for starting a raw diet also will vary from philosophical to health related and everything in between. Generally speaking, the best diet is one that makes you feel healthy and happy eating it. That could mean 100 percent raw or 75 percent raw. The trick is accepting what works for you. If you do end up eating cooked foods, make sure they are nutritious and not overly processed, such as fast food.

Don't assume raw food is a magic bullet to health. Eating a haphazard diet of raw foods could result in your being overweight or having health concerns. Too much fruit can mean too much sugar, and too many dishes that include nuts, coconut oil, and seeds can be fattening. People eating raw also can leave out too many healthful foods with no eye on balance, which can exacerbate existing health concerns or create new ones. Balance is the key.

A sensible approach is to not think in terms of restrictions. Go with foods that make you feel good physically. Raw food should make you feel strong, vibrant, and healthy, so take the time to plan your diet rather than just throwing a little lettuce and sprouts on your plate. Be mindful of what you're eating and enjoy your food. Eat a wide variety of foods with an eye on calories and getting all the nutrients required for your lifestyle.

IS PROTEIN AN ISSUE IN A RAW DIET?

People following a raw diet are often asked if they get enough protein. This could be a valid concern if the raw diet is not being followed in a sensible manner, but any diet can be nutrient deficient without variety and planning.

A well-executed raw food diet can actually exceed the daily protein recommendations of health professionals. How? Most foods, even fruit, contain some amount of protein. Protein is made up of amino acids, which are made in the body and found in food sources. The body uses protein in pretty much every task performed to keep everything running effectively. For example, proteins contract your muscles, help replace and build body tissues, transport oxygen, and convert to enzymes, antibodies, and hormones.

A complete protein is a protein that contains all nine essential amino acids. Animal source proteins are complete and complex. Plant proteins are usually incomplete, so a combination of different plant foods is required to satisfy the protein needs of the human body. There has been a great deal of research into the difference between complete and incomplete proteins, and in the past it was assumed a plant-based diet must be inferior. This is no longer considered to be true, though, with vegan and raw diets gaining acceptance in health circles. New studies have shown that incomplete proteins can be better for the body because they can be combined by the body in ways that suit its needs. Complete proteins need to be deconstructed into individual amino acids and then reconstructed. Based on research, even the recommended amount of protein thought to be necessary has dropped, and some studies show that eating animal protein increases protein needs in the body.

The best sources of protein when following a raw diet are:

Fruit

Many fruits contain complete proteins with eight amino acids. The best fruit sources of protein are usually dried fruit, such as sun-dried tomatoes, dried apricots, prunes, and raisins. Other fruits to include for protein are avocados, dates, passion fruit, tomatoes, cucumbers, and most kinds of berries.

Vegetables

While vegetables can provide some of your protein needs, it is best to combine them with other sources, such as fruits, nuts, or seeds. Good choices of protein-rich vegetables are broccoli, carrots, garlic, grape leaves, green peas, portabello mushrooms, alfalfa sprouts, brussels sprouts, and corn. Most other vegetables contain protein in smaller amounts.

Leafy Green Vegetables

This raw food staple is a wonderful way to get protein without added fat and calories. Add them to salads, drink them in smoothies, and puree them into luscious soups. Dark leafy greens to consider for your protein needs are watercress, spinach, kale, dandelion, and romaine lettuce.

Nuts and Seeds

These powerhouse little morsels are packed with protein. Many new raw food enthusiasts immediately eat a great deal of them to try to meet their daily needs. This is not a good idea. Nuts and seeds are high in fat and calories. So use nuts and seeds as an accent in most meals, combined with piles of fresh vegetables and fruits. Sprouted seeds are also a fabulous way to include protein in your diet. Good sources of protein are sunflower seeds, sesame seeds, cashews, flaxseed, chia seeds, almonds, and pumpkin seeds.

Protein Powders

Some raw food purists turn their noses up at commercially prepared protein powders. When you are first starting out, however, these products might be the best way not to fall short of your protein needs. Try to choose one that is made from raw-food-friendly sources, such as hemp, sprouted grains, or even Brazil nuts.

WHAT ARE SOME GOOD SOURCES OF NUTRIENTS IN RAW FOODS?

One of the biggest arguments against eating a raw food diet is that it is difficult to include all the required nutrients and calories. This is not true if you practice mindful eating and include a broad spectrum of foods. Here are some of the most important nutrients and the foods that contain them:

Calcium

You need calcium for strong bones, and since an ongoing issue for people who eat raw long-term is poor bone density, it is crucial to eat foods high in calcium and vitamin D. Calcium-rich foods are bok choy, almonds, sesame seeds, flaxseed, broccoli, kale, collards, endive, and figs.

Iron

Important for the blood and circulatory system, this nutrient should be eaten along with foods that contain vitamin C for better absorption. Iron-rich foods are seeds (sunflower, pumpkin, and sesame), kelp, squash, romaine lettuce, broccoli, spinach, pine nuts, cashews, and artichokes.

Magnesium

Because the refining process can strip magnesium out of processed foods, it is important to get this mineral from raw foods. Magnesium-rich foods are kale, spinach, artichokes, parsnips, almonds, cashews, pumpkin, potatoes, squash, pumpkin seeds, pine nuts, and bananas.

Zinc

A crucial element for good health, zinc helps the body produce an optimal amount of enzymes and speeds up healing. The amount of zinc in any food will usually depend on how much is in the soil the food was grown in. Good sources of zinc are seeds (chia, pumpkin, poppy, and sunflower), almonds, cashews, chard, pumpkin, avocados, bananas, and figs.

Vitamin A

This vitamin is needed to boost the immune system, promote good vision, and contribute to clear healthy skin. Good sources of vitamin A are carrots, sweet potatoes, chili powder, dark leafy greens, cantaloupe, and squash.

Vitamin B

Because raw diets often leave people deficient in vitamin B_{12}, which isn't found in plants, try taking a supplement or adding nutritional yeast to your diet. Other B vitamins (folate, riboflavin, thiamine, niacin, and panothenic acid) are found in raw food ingredients. Good sources of these vitamins are sesame seeds, sunflower seeds, pine nuts, pistachios, macadamia nuts, sun-dried tomatoes, avocados, garlic, asparagus, and hazelnuts.

Vitamin C

This powerful antioxidant is crucial for development, healing, and healthy blood vessels. Good sources of vitamin C are bell peppers, chili peppers, dark leafy greens, broccoli, kiwifruit, strawberries, and citrus fruit.

Vitamin D

Vegan and raw food diets can often be deficient in vitamin D because most of the best food sources for this vitamin are fish, seafood, and meats. Get your vitamin D requirements naturally from the sun by spending ten to fifteen minutes a day soaking it up outside. Another good source of vitamin D is mushrooms.

Vitamin E

This vitamin is actually a group of fat-soluble vitamins that help protect against some cancers, heart disease, and eye damage. Good sources of vitamin E are almonds, sunflower seeds, pine nuts, dark leafy greens, avocado, hazelnuts, papaya, and broccoli.

Vitamin K

This vitamin is absolutely essential for blood clotting and protein modification. Some good sources of vitamin K are dark leafy greens, broccoli, green onions, asparagus, and cabbage.

Essential Fatty Acids

It is very important to get enough essential fatty acids in your diet for brain function and to reduce the risk of cardiovascular disease. Good sources of essential fatty acids are flaxseed, dark leafy greens, broccoli, walnuts, sprouted radish seeds, and squash.

CAN EVERYTHING BE EATEN RAW?

Even though a plethora of raw vegetables, fruits, nuts, and sprouted seeds are undeniably healthful, some foods really should not be consumed raw, or at least not on a daily basis. Simply take a little care in your ingredient combinations, and be aware of the risks of eating the following:

- **Alfalfa sprouts.** Although these are consumed raw all the time, they do contain a toxin called canavanine, so don't eat vast quantities of these sprouts.
- **Apricot kernels.** Enjoy the succulent flesh of this stone fruit, but avoid the kernel, which contains cyanide.
- **Buckwheat.** Avoid the greens of this plant product. They can be toxic or create problems such as photosensitivity.
- **Cassava.** Some types of this plant, including the cassava flour, can be toxic.
- **Cruciferous vegetables.** These shouldn't be eaten raw constantly because they contain a chemical that can block the production of a thyroid hormone, which in time can create a hypothyroid condition. Cruciferous vegetables include cauliflower, broccoli, kale, arugula, Brussels sprouts, cabbage, and several other common vegetables.
- **Dairy.** While there are many proponents of unpasteurized milk and dairy products, pasteurization was developed for a reason. Raw dairy products can contain harmful bacteria such as *Mycobacterium bovis*, which can cause nonpulmonary tuberculosis.
- **Eggs.** Most people are aware of the possibility of salmonella in raw eggs. Salmonella can make you very sick and can even be fatal in the elderly, young children, and people with compromised immune systems.
- **Kidney beans.** Eaten raw, the sprouts and beans can be toxic because they contain a chemical called phytohaemagglutinin.
- **Meat.** Raw meat can be a fertile environment for viruses, bacteria, and parasites.
- **Peas.** Some types of raw peas of one genus (*Lathyrus*) can cause neurological problems in the lower legs if consumed raw.
- **Potatoes.** Raw potatoes contain hemagglutinins, which reduce effective red blood cell function.
- **Rhubarb.** While the stalks of this plant can be eaten raw, they are better when dehydrated for several hours on the higher temperature end.

The leaves of the rhubarb plant, however, are poisonous and should never be eaten.

- **Vegetable greens.** Eat these in moderation because many greens contain oxalic acid, which can contribute to the formation of kidney stones and block the absorption of calcium and iron.

IS A RAW FOOD DIET SAFE FOR EVERYONE?

Anyone wishing to start a new eating plan or a restricted diet of any kind should consult a medical professional to go over the risks and discuss if the diet is safe. It is also a good idea to conduct a great deal of research on the diet. Many diets fail or become dangerous when people do not plan carefully to get the right amount of nutrients and calories to function. Keep in mind that even if you get a green light from your doctor and have a comprehensive path to follow, you should still avoid starting a 100 percent raw diet, because your body might not be able to handle it. If you are someone who eats meat three or four times a week, drinks a lot of coffee, or has a sweet tooth, you could experience overwhelmingly uncomfortable symptoms and cravings with such a drastic change. Take your time and build up to a predominantly raw diet.

A true raw diet is not safe without proper planning. This diet takes a certain commitment to preparation and well-thought-out meals to ensure you don't end up with a nutritional deficiency. Eating your favorite salad every day for all your meals is not what this diet is meant to be, even if your salad is raw. The best way to stay healthy is to eat a vast variety of foods, all the colors and types possible. Some studies indicate the need to be particularly careful about calcium, vitamin D, and vitamin B_{12} on a raw diet. Deficiencies in these can cause dangerously low bone density, a weak immune system, impaired cognitive function, and anemia.

If you have other health issues, you might have to commit to a lower percentage of raw food to ensure you don't put your health at risk. The following are some of the conditions that make this a poor diet choice.

Eating Disorders

Eating disorders create an obsession with food that can be transferred to a raw-food-diet doctrine. People with eating disorders are also prone to malnutrition, so a poorly planned raw diet could be as dangerous as not eating or purging.

Young Children

There are families with young children who follow a completely raw diet, but these are usually people who have been living raw for a long time with a great deal of knowledge and practical experience. The risk with kids comes when the diet is too restrictive, is not varied enough, and excludes important nutrients required for growth and development. When in doubt, consult your pediatrician and perhaps try for a limited raw food diet.

Diabetes and Hypoglycemia

A well-planned, comprehensive raw diet can be quite healthful for people with these conditions. Unfortunately, many people without good raw cookbooks or enough information start their raw diet by eating a great deal of fruit. This large intake of natural sugar can create blood sugar issues and exacerbate hypoglycemic symptoms.

CHAPTER FIVE

The Health and Weight-Loss Benefits of a Raw Diet

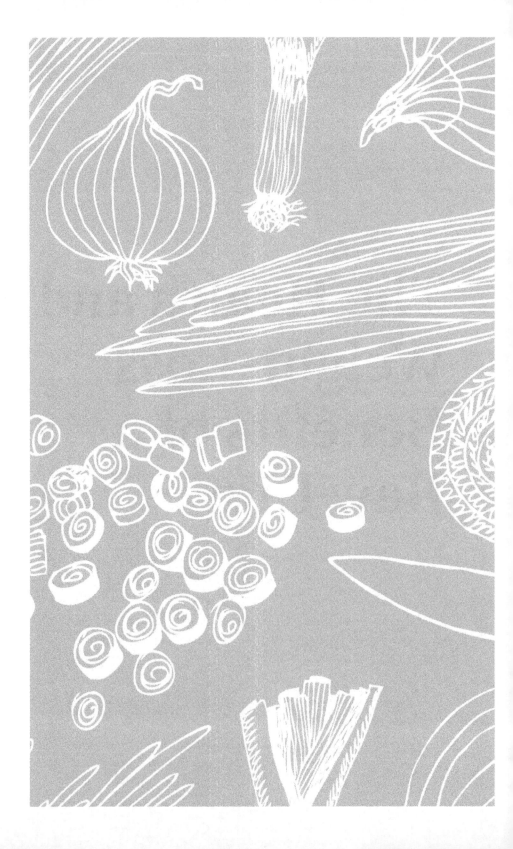

The Health and Weight-Loss Benefits of a Raw Diet

People start a raw food diet for many different reasons. The majority, however, do it to improve general well-being or to address an existing health concern. Raw food is often thought to be a natural means to treat health issues, with the goal of perhaps eventually curing the problem. Whatever the reason for trying raw foods, some real benefits are seen even during the diet's transition phase.

CAN EATING RAW IMPROVE YOUR HEALTH?

Unfortunately, there is not a great deal of research yet about the raw food diet. Since it is gaining in popularity, that might change in the near future. Most conclusions and statistics are derived from vegan and vegetarian studies. There are many simple reasons why raw food can produce so many health benefits. One just has to look at the ingredients people eat when following a well-planned raw diet to see a logical connection to vibrant, glowing health.

One recommended strategy for better health long touted by health professionals is eating a large quantity of fresh produce every day. Most people in developed countries eat about three servings of fruits and vegetables a day, whereas people eating raw typically have eighteen servings in the same time frame. This makes a huge difference. Raw foods are very high in fiber, nutrients, and phytochemicals and low in saturated fats, sodium, cholesterol, and refined sugars. They do not contain harmful additives, preservatives, or dyes and are not prepared using unhealthful techniques, such as deep-fat frying or barbecuing. Raw foods are also on the low acid side of the alkaline–acid scale. This is beneficial because studies have shown too much acidity in the body can contribute to disease.

WHAT ARE THE HEALTH BENEFITS OF EATING RAW?

When you start to eat raw, the first thing you might notice is a little extra spring in your step. Increased and sustained energy levels are definitely a benefit. That midafternoon slump will be a thing of the past, and all you will need is a little fruit to provide a quick recharge. On top of this increased energy, you might also notice you sleep better and need less sleep to be perky all day. Very likely, you'll wake up without feeling groggy and tired.

Along with all that energy, most raw foodists report less mental fog. You might be able to focus longer and with more clarity throughout the day. This sharpening of the mind could be due to the energy boost, or it might be connected to less toxin buildup in the body. Either way, you can devote your mind to things that are important and stay alert while doing so. This mental clarity can often have a positive impact on mood as well, so don't be surprised to find yourself smiling more.

Another benefit of eating raw is an improvement in skin appearance and tone. One of the misassumptions made about skin is that problems such as acne and dullness are skin deep. Diet has a huge impact on skin, and your skin will often reflect what's going on inside your body. Our skin is usually the last organ to get nutrients, because it isn't a vital organ. This means if your diet is deficient, your skin is left without vitamins, minerals, and other nutrients to repair damage and thrive. Typical fat-laden processed foods can clog capillaries and produce metabolic waste, creating acne and in the long run aging the skin prematurely. Raw food provides an overabundance of vital nutrients without the harmful elements. The result? Skin that simply blooms with health.

One of the most important health considerations when eating a raw food diet is a significant lowering of LDL or "bad" cholesterol, triglycerides, system-wide inflammation, and blood sugar levels in the body. This means a reduction in the risk of developing cardiovascular disease and diabetes. An October 2012 report in *Food Technology* connects eating plant-based diets with a reduction or outright elimination of the genetic predisposition to developing type 2 diabetes, cardiovascular disease, and cancer. This reason alone should convince people to at least try a diet made up of 75 percent raw foods.

Cancer has been the focus of many diet-based research projects, and raw foods are a lifestyle choice of great interest to many scientists. A raw food diet has been found to reduce the risk of many types of cancers, including prostate, bladder, laryngeal, oral, gastric, and breast cancers. Even adding just one raw meal a day can impact your risk for certain types of cancers.

Everyone will experience different health benefits from eating raw, because we all start the diet at unique physical conditions and approach the transition and execution of the plan differently. With this in mind, other ailments documented to be positively influenced by a raw food diet are:

- Allergies
- Arthritis
- Asthma
- Back, neck, and joint pain
- Candida
- Chronic fatigue
- Colitis
- Depression and anxiety
- Diverticulitis
- Excessive or painful menstruation
- Fibromyalgia
- Heartburn
- Migraines

WEIGHT LOSS AND RAW FOOD

One of the most common reasons people start a raw food diet is to lose weight. Dropping excess pounds can also be the foundation for reducing the risk of many serious conditions, such as diabetes and cardiovascular disease. Whether losing weight is the goal or a pleasant side effect, it is easy to see why it happens on this plan. Consuming huge quantities of fresh, healthful produce while eliminating fatty, sugar-laden processed foods is a sure path to a lower body mass index (BMI). Coincidentally or not, in most cases people eating raw do have a healthful or low BMI.

Cooking techniques often add calories, fat, sodium, and sugar to a finished dish. Think of braising in rich sauces, butter melting in a skillet to fry eggs, or how much oil is absorbed when foods are deep-fried. Just eliminating the cooking step can create a diet that practically guarantees weight loss. Also consider that raw foods are not usually calorie dense. This means you can fill up on vegetables, fruits, and seeds without exceeding your daily calorie requirements. All that fiber and water in raw foods also contributes to weight loss because they help your digestion work more effectively to purge system-clogging waste.

Can you gain weight eating raw? The raw diet might seem like a magic bullet for slimming down, but it cannot circumvent the time-tested rule of what happens when more calories are consumed than expended. Those excess calories, whether from French fries or almond butter, will be converted to body fat. Keep a close eye on your nut, nut butter, and seed consumption. Although nuts and seeds are nutrient-packed, they are also high in fat. This is when balance and planning come into play. Keep your menu packed with produce, and use nuts or seeds to provide taste and texture.

CHAPTER SIX

Beginning Your Transition to a Raw Food Diet

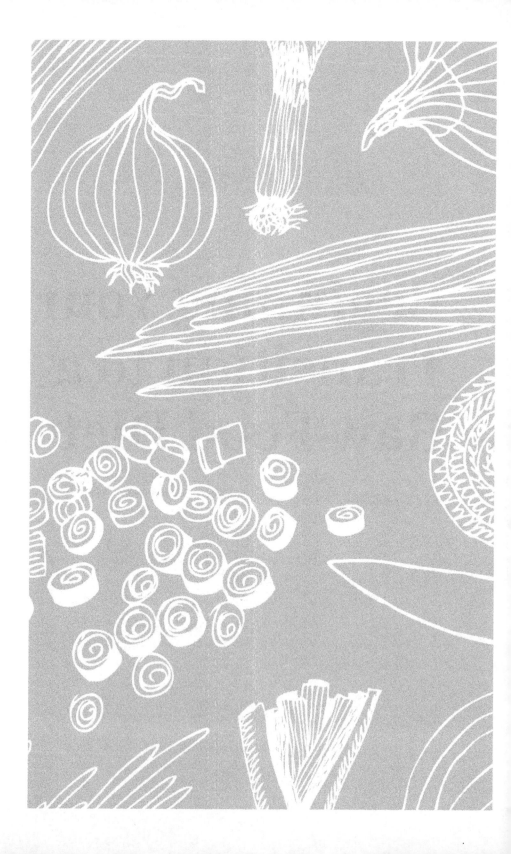

Beginning Your Transition to a Raw Food Diet

WHAT KIND OF EATING HABITS DO YOU HAVE?

To determine the best way to transition to raw foods, take a close, hard look at your eating habits. A good relationship with food is crucial when embarking on this type of lifestyle change.

1. How many caffeinated beverages do you drink per day?
2. Do you have one or more alcoholic beverages per day?
3. How many spoonfuls of sugar do you add to your beverages and food each day?
4. Do you eat a great deal of breads or grains?
5. How many servings of fruits and vegetables do you eat per day?
6. What kind of snacks do you eat?
7. Do you eat breakfast?
8. Do you eat when depressed, bored, or upset?
9. How often do you read food labels?
10. Do you have a good understanding of healthful eating principles?
11. Do you eat every two to three hours throughout the day or eat three big meals?
12. Do you eat a variety of foods each day?
13. Has your weight changed in the last six months? If so, how?
14. Has your health changed in the last six months?
15. Do you sit down to eat or do you eat on the run?
16. How often do you eat vegetarian meals?

If you eat a great deal of sugar or caffeine, you may find you need a slower transition to a raw diet to avoid withdrawal symptoms. When you look at your diet you might see many items found on the raw diet or you might notice that there are very few features in common. If your diet is already predominantly vegetables and fruits eaten frequently throughout the day with little or no added sugar, you might be able to jump to 75 percent raw without any issues.

WHAT SHOULD BE IN A RAW FOOD PANTRY, AND WHAT SHOULD BE THROWN AWAY?

A big fear of new raw foodists is that they will be consuming raw salads for the rest of their lives. This is not quite true. You will be enjoying an assortment of tempting salads filled with exotic and familiar ingredients, but you also will be trying tasty wraps, simple vegetable pastas, and even desserts. The trick of a successful raw food diet is to try a broad range of different foods to avoid culinary burnout and nutritional deficiencies.

Foods You Should Have in Your Pantry and Refrigerator

Whether your diet consists of 75 percent or up to 100 percent raw food, staples of the basic raw food diet include:

- Carob powder and raw cacao nibs
- Fresh juices
- Fruits and dried fruits (from a reputable raw supplier)
- Herbs, spices, and condiments
- Nuts and seeds (including nut milks, flours, and butters)
- Oils (raw coconut oil, coconut butter, extra-virgin olive oil)
- Organic and air-dried spices
- Protein powder (raw)
- Raw (not heat-cultured) miso, nama shoyu, kimchee, and sauerkraut
- Raw sweeteners (honey, agave nectar, maple syrup, and coconut nectar)
- Sea vegetables and seaweed
- Some naturally dried legumes
- Sprouted seeds and grains
- Vegetables
- Whole raw grains and pulses

Some raw food enthusiasts eat animal products as well, but you must find these from reputable sources. Raw animal products that might be included are raw milk, organic eggs, beef, fish, and raw-milk cheeses.

Foods You Should Clear Out of Your Pantry and Refrigerator

The following ingredients and products should be banished only if you have committed to 100 percent raw food eating. If you are simply trying for a lower percentage of raw food, then some of these items can be eaten at least part of the time. Whenever you can, eat simply prepared fresh foods that are as close to their natural form as possible.

- **Alcohol and caffeine.** These items are also a personal choice for many people, but they do not belong on most raw food diets. Some red wines, however, have the right criteria to be considered raw. Do your homework, and you might find a gem to enjoy with your dinner.
- **Cooked foods.** Since eating raw is all about keeping your food below 118 degrees F, cooked foods are not supposed to make their way to your plate. This includes canned foods and some dried foods.
- **Cooked grains and legumes.** This food group is where vegans and raw foodists part ways. Vegans eat many grains, breads, and legumes, whereas those following the raw food diet eat only some sprouted varieties.
- **Processed foods.** Anything that has ingredients you cannot recognize or pronounce is off the menu in the raw food diet. Products containing refined flours, sugars, and additives should also be avoided.
- **Soy and meat alternatives.** Tofu and soy products are often processed at higher temperatures than are allowed on a raw food diet. If you're not eating 100 percent raw, tofu can be a smart choice for your "cooked" percentage because it is compatible with many of the other ingredients enjoyed on the raw diet.
- **Sugar.** Many raw food enthusiasts avoid sugars in any form. It's a personal choice whether you want to include items such as maple syrup, honey, or agave nectar. Obviously, refined sugars and artificial sweeteners are off-limits in any healthful diet.

EQUIPMENT AND TOOLS

While you can create many wonderful raw food recipes with just a good knife and a cutting board, some basic cooking tools will make your life easier and meals more convenient. Raw food recipes often include these tools because they create diversity and interesting textures. Some preparations include dehydrating, sprouting, juicing, blending, chopping, pureeing, and soaking. Some of the equipment and kitchen tools to consider for your raw food adventures are:

- **Blender or immersion blender.** If you don't have a food processor or juicer, then a blender is an essential tool for raw eating. An immersion blender is a convenient handheld tool that you can use for less heavy-duty processing tasks.
- **Dehydrator.** If you are serious about committing to a raw food diet, a quality dehydrator is a necessity. You don't have to purchase one right away, but it will increase the variety of recipes you can try.
- **Food processor.** Leave this indispensible tool out on your counter. A processor can chop vegetables, puree soups and sauces, make dough for desserts, and is essential for nut butters, flours, and milks.
- **Juicer.** You could probably do without having a juicer on a raw diet, but why limit your choices? Many soups, sauces, and smoothies require juiced products as a base for the finished dish.
- **Mandoline.** Used to create julienned vegetables, crinkle cuts, ribbons, and batons, this tool can be tricky to use, but with a little practice you can safely process piles of tasty produce.
- **Nesting bowls.** Invest in quality stainless steel products in different sizes.
- **Quality chef's knives.** Even if you have the best-stocked, most modern kitchen in the world, you will still be chopping, dicing, and mincing a great deal of produce with a simple knife. Invest in several professional-caliber knives to make this task simpler and safer. Professional knives are better balanced, sharper, and last longer. Consider buying an assortment to suit your needs, such as paring knives, a cleaver, and a basic knife. Take the time to hold each knife to feel how it fits your hand. Each size and brand will be very different.
- **Sealable, stackable containers.** Correct storage of raw food is important to avoid spoilage. They also come in handy for soaking and sprouting beans and grains.

- **Specialized tools.** You might not need a tool to section your grapefruits or core your apples, but they certainly make meal preparation easier. Quite a few small chef's tools come in handy when preparing raw food, so pick up a few along with your new knives. Some good choices to have are a vegetable peeler, a grapefruit knife, an apple corer, a melon baller, a zester, a grater, and a channel knife.
- **Thermometer.** Find a high-quality digital thermometer that reads low numbers. That way you'll be confident that your food is in the correct range for the raw diet.
- **Wet and dry measuring cups.** These must-have items ensure the success of the finished product.

15 TIPS FOR TRANSITIONING TO A RAW FOOD DIET

- **Research, research, and more research.** For you to follow a healthful and satisfying diet, the best tool to have is knowledge. The raw food diet requires knowing what to eat, why you should eat it, and how much to eat. Before embarking on this culinary journey, read lots of books, visit the many websites that can educate you about this diet, and visit a local raw food restaurant to sample the food.
- **Get ready to answer questions.** Don't be surprised if at first the people in your life are not enthusiastic about your choice to go raw. There will be questions, so be prepared to answer them. For example, are you eating raw to lose weight? What is a raw diet? Articulate your reasons clearly, and don't let their questions discourage you.
- **Accept your starting point.** You might be a practicing vegan who jogs every day or someone whose idea of exercise and healthful eating is getting off the couch to grab a bag of potato chips. It doesn't matter where you are starting raw from, just that you are making the change.
- **Just try the diet.** At some point you will have to stop researching the diet and start it. Don't let ambiguity about the scientific doctrine behind raw foods or the unfamiliarity of the ingredients keep you from incorporating a few raw foods into your daily routine. Give the diet your best shot, and see if this eating plan fits your palate and your lifestyle.
- **Eliminate processed foods.** The simplest way to transition quickly to raw foods is to ban processed food from your diet. Consider your eating habits before taking a cold-turkey approach to foods such as sweets or coffee. If

you are a sugar junkie, cutting out sweets could create such serious detox symptoms as headaches and nausea. Replace the processed items with approved raw alternatives whenever possible, such as maple syrup or agave nectar. When you go shopping, your cart should have a minimum of packaged items. When considering if a product is processed, a good rule of thumb is to read the label for additives and lengthy lists of unpronounceable ingredients.

- **Find recipes that are easy to prepare, and talk to people who eat raw.** Nothing can derail a new diet faster than not understanding recipe directions, not recognizing ingredients, or being unfamiliar with the spices of the dish. Begin by following recipes that use ingredients found in your usual market and equipment that you already own. Once you become more familiar with the diet, you can branch out and experiment. It also might be helpful to talk to people who are already on this culinary path. You can find out the best places to shop, how to overcome some of the challenges, and even swap recipes. There are countless physical and virtual raw food communities to join, so take a look around and find one that suits you.

- **Understand the correct way to prepare and store foods.** Because they spoil more quickly, raw foods need to be handled a little differently than cooked or processed foods. You will need to prepare your raw foods quite frequently to ensure food safety and freshness. You can freeze some raw foods such as coconut, grains, nuts, and dried fruit to keep them fresh for as long as possible. Always follow the recipes closely with respect to storage (refrigerator or room temperature) so the finished dish is the best it can be.

- **Plan everything.** There is an old saying about failing to plan and planning to fail, which is appropriate when transitioning to raw. If you "wing" this diet, you could do damage to yourself, especially if 100 percent raw is your goal. Take the time to create a comprehensive menu plan for yourself, including preparation times. Start a food journal so you know exactly what you are eating and where you need to fill in your nutrition gaps. This will put you on the right path to understanding the concept of mindful eating as well.

- **Eat a variety of foods.** This is probably the most important thing to remember when transitioning to a raw food diet because your health could depend on it. The more color and types of foods on your plate, the more likely you will meet and exceed your nutritional needs. When starting your raw food diet, make a list of all the ingredients you like that are found in raw food preparation. Expand it with ingredients you have seen at your local store. Plan a few days of menus. Eat even one meal that is totally raw and work your way up from there, including more meals using the ingredients on your list. To provide variety, try different preparation techniques as well. Keep in mind that you will need to become very familiar with spices and herbs to make your raw meals taste complex. Think about your favorite foods, and see if you can make a raw version. For example, with a little practice, apple crumble is quite easy to re-create raw. Pasta, often a favorite family meal, can be transformed by pouring a tasty fresh tomato sauce over vegetable noodles or kelp noodles.

- **Understand that habits are hard to break.** There are going to be times when you forget why you want to follow a raw lifestyle, because it is easier to eat what you are used to eating. Convenience foods are, well, convenient. What is simpler than microwaving a can of soup or picking up a toasted bagel from your favorite diner? Understanding that you are following a routine that you set up yourself can make it easier to create new routines that feature raw food. Eventually, reaching for a donut when you're feeling blue will no longer be a habit. Instead, taking a walk while chomping on a crunchy apple will.

- **Do not overspend when eating raw.** Spending a fortune to follow a raw diet can be discouraging. If you are independently wealthy, then this might not be a concern, but most people have to live within a budget. At first glance it might look like you are outlaying a fair amount of money for all your fresh produce, seeds, nuts, and other exotic ingredients, especially if you are buying organic. This could be the case, but compared dollar for dollar, the healthful nutrient-packed food in your grocery cart is much better value than the empty calories of the processed foods that might have been there previously. Try to find local farmers' markets where fresh fruits and vegetables can be found at a fraction of the price. Buy in bulk whenever possible and stay away from ingredients that you have no idea how to prepare or you might end up wasting them.

- **Understand that this diet might take more time to prepare.** Some raw food dishes are easy to create and others have to be done over the course of hours, sometimes over a day, depending on the recipe. If you want to serve a hearty chili made from dehydrated vegetables and a fresh tomato sauce, be aware that you need to start it before you leave the house at breakfast time, not after work about an hour before dinner. Dehydrating in particular can be a lengthy process.

- **Start by being a vegan.** This is often a good training-wheels step to eating raw, because there are so many vegan versions of favorite foods available even in mainstream grocery stores. You can even find vegan bacon and baked products. Once you have transitioned to a cooked vegan diet successfully, take another step to a raw diet. The detox from vegan to raw is also almost nonexistent, and because you can still eat most of your vegan favorites, you might not find yourself missing any foods at all.

- **You should never feel worse eating raw.** After you recover from the headaches and other common physical ailments experienced while transitioning to a raw diet, you should feel pretty good. Depending on the state of your diet before eating raw, you might feel significantly better, and if you don't, something is amiss. Take a thorough look at what you are eating to make sure you are covering your nutrition bases. If you are, it might be time to visit your doctor. A well-planned, comprehensive raw diet should give you energy, a sparkle in your eye, shiny locks, and a positive outlook.

- **Cut yourself some slack.** Although eating raw is more of a lifestyle choice than a diet, the same rules apply to raw eating as to any other eating plan. If you fall off the wagon, don't be consumed with guilt or take it as a reason to blow the wagon up, so to speak. You might eat something that is not raw. You might eat something so far removed from raw it might survive a bomb blast. That is okay. It is only food and what you eat is ultimately your own choice. Have a glass of wine every once in a while if you enjoy it and understand your raw experience is your own. Make educated choices, be healthy, be vibrant, and enjoy life.

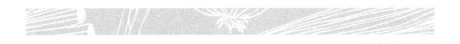

CHAPTER SEVEN

Breakfasts

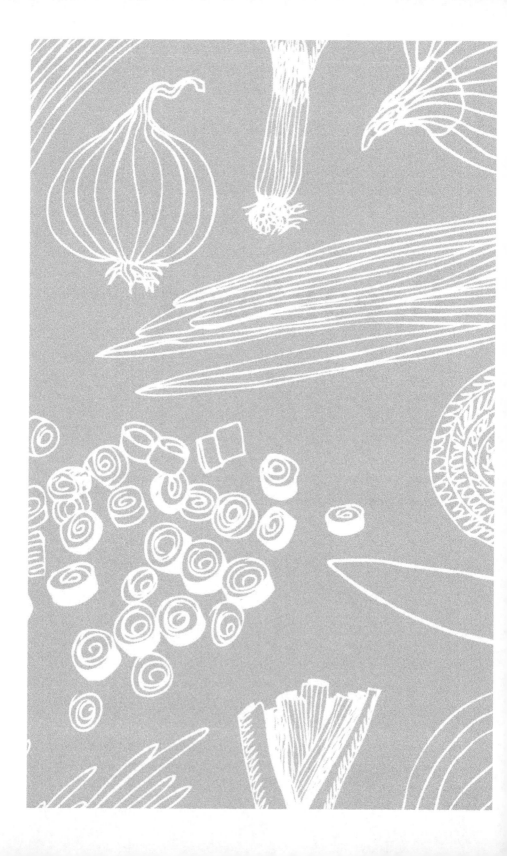

Mixed Berry Banana Crepes

MAKES 4–6 SERVINGS

Except for the color, these crepes look a lot like their French-style counterparts. The trick to this lovely dish is to watch the crepes carefully and remove them from the dehydrator as soon as they are dry enough to pick up and still pliable enough to roll easily. You can use almost any fruit as a filling. Try peaches, spiced apples, and even mango for delicious variations.

FOR THE CREPES:
5 LARGE RIPE BANANAS, PEELED
JUICE OF 1 LEMON

FOR THE VANILLA CREAM AND BERRIES:
1 CUP CASHEWS, SOAKED IN WATER FOR AT LEAST 6 HOURS, RINSED, AND DRAINED
MEAT FROM 2 SMALL COCONUTS
2 TEASPOONS AGAVE NECTAR
1 TABLESPOON PURE VANILLA EXTRACT
4 CUPS MIXED BERRIES

Make the crepes:

1. Put the bananas in a blender with the lemon juice, and process until smooth and liquid.

2. Pour the banana mixture into 6-inch circles about 1/8 inch thick on dehydrator sheets covered in nonstick pads.

3. Dehydrate for 6–8 hours at 115 degrees F until flexible but not overly dry.

Make the vanilla cream and berries:

1. Place all the ingredients except the berries in a blender and process until smooth. Transfer the mixture to a small bowl and chill in the refrigerator to thicken.

2. Place two crepes on a plate and spoon vanilla cream onto half of each crepe. Top the vanilla cream with berries and fold the crepes over.

Banana Nut Pancakes

Pancakes are a wonderful way to start the day, especially on a lazy Sunday morning. The combination of banana and pecan in this recipe is traditional and creates an almost toasty flavor. If you skip the maple syrup, these pancakes are a convenient snack to eat plain on the run. The initial stage in the dehydrator uses a higher temperature than what is usually recommended for raw food, but since the pancakes never reach that temperature, it is okay.

2 CUPS GROUND FLAXSEED

2 LARGE BANANAS, PEELED AND SLICED

1 CUP WATER

1 CUP CHOPPED PECANS

⅔ CUP UNSWEETENED SHREDDED COCONUT

⅔ CUP FLAXSEED

⅓ CUP COCONUT BUTTER, SOFTENED

⅓ CUP PURE MAPLE SYRUP, WITH EXTRA FOR TOPPING

1. Use your hands to combine all the ingredients except the maple syrup in a large bowl until well mixed. Shape the mixture into pancakes, about ½ inch thick and 5 inches in diameter.

2. Place the pancakes on dehydrator screens and dehydrate at 140 degrees F for 45 minutes. Reduce the heat to 115 degrees F and dehydrate for 30 minutes.

3. Top with maple syrup or eat plain.

Rice Pudding

MAKES 6 SERVINGS

This is simple, satisfying comfort food. The white chia seeds swell up, creating a look and texture very close to traditional rice pudding. While you can make this pudding with black chia seeds, the dish will not be as appealing. The pudding will appear grayish instead of white, but will taste similar.

1 CUP CASHEWS, SOAKED IN WATER FOR 10 HOURS,
    RINSED, AND DRAINED
2 CUPS ALMOND MILK (SEE RECIPE IN CHAPTER 12)
2 TABLESPOONS PURE MAPLE SYRUP
SEEDS FROM 1 VANILLA BEAN, SCRAPED OUT
1 TABLESPOON PURE VANILLA EXTRACT
1 TEASPOON GROUND CINNAMON
PINCH OF SEA SALT
⅓ CUP WHITE CHIA SEEDS

1. Place all the ingredients except the chia seeds in a blender, and process until completely smooth.

2. Pour the mixture into a large bowl and stir in the chia seeds.

3. Cover the bowl and chill in the refrigerator for 4–10 hours.

4. Serve chilled.

Apple Oatmeal

This versatile dish can be made with many different kinds of fruits and spices. You can even put it through a blender to create a creamier texture. Oats contain all the major nutrient groups required by the body. Some people are sensitive to the phytic acid in this grain. If you are one of them, always soak your oats overnight with a little salt and then drain them in the morning, rinsing well.

2 CUPS ALMOND MILK (SEE RECIPE IN CHAPTER 12)

1 CUP OLD-FASHIONED ROLLED OATS

⅓ CUP APPLE BUTTER

2 TABLESPOONS AGAVE NECTAR

½ TEASPOON GROUND CINNAMON

2 TABLESPOONS CHOPPED ALMONDS

1 LARGE TART APPLE, DICED, FOR GARNISH

1. In a large bowl stir together the almond milk, rolled oats, apple butter, agave nectar, and cinnamon until well combined.

2. Cover the bowl and place in the refrigerator overnight. Adjust the thickness with a little more almond milk if desired.

3. Top with chopped almonds and diced apple.

Old-Fashioned Applesauce

This simple, unadorned applesauce is as close to biting into an apple as you can get. If you are looking for a smoother applesauce, remove the apple skins. Leave the skins for a finished dish that will have more texture, a slightly rosy color (if you use red apples), and more nutrients. Apple skin contains soluble and insoluble fiber, pectin, quercetin, and antioxidants.

1 CUP WATER, OR AS NEEDED

⅔ CUP PITTED DATES

8 LARGE APPLES, CORED AND CHOPPED ROUGHLY

¼ CUP FRESH LEMON JUICE

1 TEASPOON GROUND CINNAMON

¼ TEASPOON GROUND NUTMEG

1. Place the water and dates in a small bowl, and soak them for about 1 hour until soft. Drain, reserving the water.

2. Transfer the dates to a food processor with the apples and about ⅓ cup of the reserved water, and pulse a few times.

3. Add the lemon juice and spices, and pulse until it achieves the consistency you want. Adjust the seasonings if necessary and serve.

4. The applesauce can be stored in the refrigerator for 3–4 days.

Honey Granola

MAKES 8 CUPS

This is the last granola recipe you will ever need, because it is the best. You can use this granola on a vast assortment of dishes to impart texture, flavor, and nutritional benefits. Make a double batch so you will always have some on hand. This recipe can be adjusted to suit your taste, so feel free to add different nuts, seeds, and dried fruits.

6 CUPS OLD-FASHIONED ROLLED OATS
1½ CUPS UNSWEETENED SHREDDED COCONUT
1 CUP SUNFLOWER SEEDS
1 CUP SLICED ALMONDS
1 CUP RAISINS
½ CUP PUMPKIN SEEDS
½ CUP HAZELNUTS
½ CUP DRIED CRANBERRIES
1 TEASPOON GROUND CINNAMON
½ TEASPOON GROUND NUTMEG
½ CUP RAW HONEY
⅓ CUP EXTRA-VIRGIN OLIVE OIL

1. In a large bowl toss together all the ingredients except the honey and olive oil, and mix well.

2. In a small bowl stir together the honey and olive oil until well blended.

3. Pour the honey mixture into the oat mixture. Use your hands to toss the mixture until well coated.

4. Transfer the mixture to four dehydrator sheets, and dehydrate for 4–6 hours at 110 degrees F or until very dry. Stir the mixture every hour or so.

5. Store the granola in airtight containers in the refrigerator or freezer.

Morning Energy Bars

MAKES 16 BARS

Hectic mornings call for a quick, ready-made bar. These energy bars are a nutritious way to start a busy day and are very simple to put together. You can even double the batch and store the extras in the freezer until you need them. Simply let them thaw in the refrigerator overnight so they aren't too hard in the morning.

1 CUP PITTED DATES

1 CUP PECANS

1 CUP PUMPKIN SEEDS

½ CUP DRIED CRANBERRIES

½ CUP UNSWEETENED SHREDDED COCONUT

⅓ CUP CHIA SEEDS

⅓ CUP GROUND FLAXSEED

¼ CUP CACAO NIBS

¼ CUP HEMP SEEDS

2 TABLESPOONS MELTED COCONUT OIL, IF NEEDED

1. Line a 9 × 13–inch baking dish with parchment paper and set aside.

2. Combine all the ingredients except the coconut oil in a food processor, and pulse until everything sticks together.

3. If the mixture seems too dry, add the melted coconut oil as needed.

4. Press the mixture into the prepared baking dish, and place in the refrigerator for about 2 hours.

5. Cut the chilled bars into 16 equal pieces.

6. Store the bars in a container in the refrigerator.

Vanilla Cream with Peaches

MAKES 4 SERVINGS

Start your day with a smile with this tasty combination. Don't despair if at first your cream isn't smooth. This process takes a little time, especially if your blender is not a heavy-duty commercial product. Try pulsing your ingredients before putting the blender on high speed, and make sure you chop everything up into small pieces. Instead of peaches, you can serve this dish with other fruits, such as berries.

4 CUPS FRESH CHOPPED COCONUT MEAT

16 DATES, PITTED

⅓ CUP CASHEWS, SOAKED IN WATER FOR 8–10 HOURS, RINSED, AND DRAINED

⅓ CUP COCONUT WATER

SEEDS FROM 1 VANILLA BEAN, SCRAPED OUT

1 TEASPOON PURE VANILLA EXTRACT

4 LARGE RIPE PEACHES, PITTED AND SLICED

1. Place all the ingredients except the peaches in a blender, and process until smooth and creamy.

2. Transfer to a bowl and chill.

3. Serve with the sliced peaches.

Lemon Curd
with Blackberries

MAKES 4 SERVINGS

This tart, smooth treat is like eating dessert for breakfast. The coconut in the recipe is a nutritional superstar, and it will give you a great deal of energy to start the day. It can boost energy and endurance while improving your digestion. When you add those benefits to cashews, which promote energy production, you have a powerhouse dish.

1 CUP CASHEWS, SOAKED IN WATER FOR 8 HOURS,
    RINSED, AND DRAINED
⅔ CUP FRESH CHOPPED COCONUT MEAT
JUICE AND ZEST OF 3 LEMONS
⅓ CUP WATER
⅔ CUP AGAVE NECTAR, TO TASTE
SEA SALT TO TASTE
4 CUPS RIPE BLACKBERRIES

1. Place the cashews, coconut, lemon juice, lemon zest, and water in a food processor and blend until creamy and smooth.

2. Add the agave nectar and blend until well incorporated.

3. Add the sea salt and transfer the lemon curd to a sealable container.

4. Place the curd in the refrigerator, sealed, until you are ready to serve it.

5. Spoon the curd into serving bowls and top with the blackberries.

Almond Cranberry Bread

MAKES 20 PIECES

If you make your own almond milk, this recipe is a terrific way to use up the almond flour left in the cheesecloth. This bread is more biscotti-like than soft, and you need to score the dough quite deeply to create neat square pieces. You will find this bread absolutely sublime dunked in a cup of herbal tea or a glass of almond milk.

6 CUPS ALMOND FLOUR

1½ CUPS DRIED CRANBERRIES

1 CUP GROUND FLAXSEED

1⅓ CUPS EXTRA-VIRGIN OLIVE OIL OR COCONUT OIL

1 TEASPOON SEA SALT

1. Combine the almond flour, cranberries, and ground flaxseed in a large bowl.

2. Add the olive oil and salt, and mix well with your hands until a dough forms.

3. Press the almond dough firmly onto a drying sheet until it is uniformly ¼ inch thick.

4. Use a sharp knife to score the dough into 20 pieces.

5. Place another dehydrator sheet directly on top of the bread and flip the sheets over.

6. Remove the top dehydrator sheet.

7. Dehydrate for 7–8 hours at 105 degrees F.

CHAPTER EIGHT

Soups

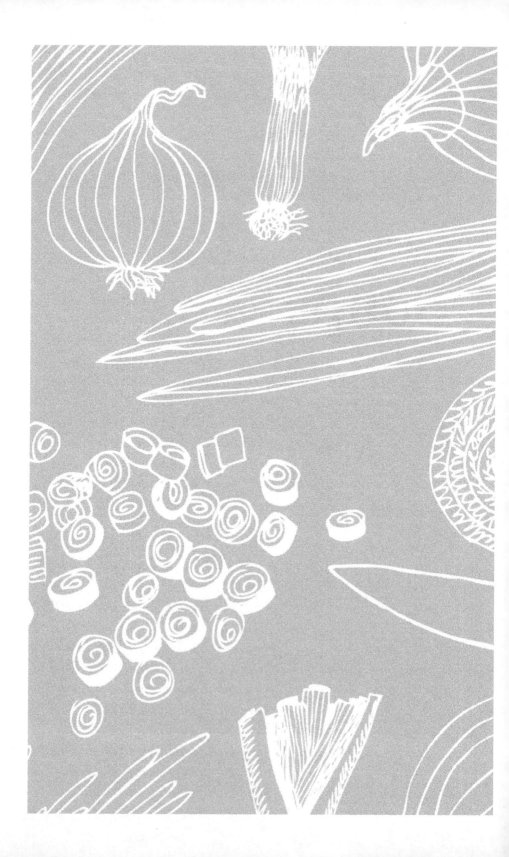

Avocado Lime Soup

Imagine the most delicate pale green color dappled with darker fresh green flecks of chives, and that will be pretty close to this soup. Incredibly fresh, it has a satisfying creaminess. This is a perfect summer soup to serve to friends and family.

4 AVOCADOS, PEELED AND PITTED

1 MEDIUM CUCUMBER, WASHED, WITH THE SKIN ON

2 STALKS CELERY

JUICE OF 2 LIMES

¼ CUP FRESH CHOPPED CILANTRO

2 TABLESPOONS GROUND CUMIN

1 TABLESPOON GROUND CORIANDER

1 TABLESPOON TAMARI

2 CUPS WATER

1 TEASPOON SEA SALT, OR TO TASTE

FRESHLY GROUND BLACK PEPPER, TO TASTE

CHOPPED CHIVES AND RAW SOUR CREAM
(SEE RECIPE IN CHAPTER 12), FOR GARNISH

1. Place all the ingredients except the sea salt, black pepper, and garnish in a large blender and pulse until very smooth.

2. Season the soup with the sea salt and black pepper to taste.

3. Transfer the soup to serving bowls and garnish.

Celeriac Soup

Ever come across celeriac in the grocery store and wonder how this bumpy root ball is used in recipes? Celeriac, a fresh, firm-textured root vegetable, can be a staple ingredient in soups and many other dishes because it combines well with a long list of ingredients. This soup is quite thick when it is finished and will take some extra time to get smooth. If you'd like to speed the process along, try cutting the celeriac into very small pieces.

3 CELERIAC BULBS, PEELED AND CHOPPED

5 CELERY STALKS, CHOPPED

½ SMALL SWEET ONION

4 CUPS WATER

JUICE FROM 1 LEMON

¼ CUP EXTRA-VIRGIN OLIVE OIL

SEA SALT AND FRESHLY GROUND BLACK PEPPER, TO TASTE

1. Place all the ingredients in a blender and process until smooth.

2. Pour the soup through a mesh sieve and adjust the seasonings.

Elegant Shiitake Mushroom Soup

Shiitake mushrooms have an earthy, meaty flavor that comes as a surprise when sampling this delicate, golden broth-based soup. To extract as much of the mushroom flavor as possible from the soaked mushrooms, squeeze the mushrooms against the sieve when draining off the liquid. This soup could also be dressed up with other herbs and minced baby carrots or a hint of garlic.

6 CUPS DRIED SHIITAKE MUSHROOMS
10 CUPS WATER
2 TABLESPOONS NAMA SHOYU
SEA SALT AND FRESHLY GROUND BLACK PEPPER, TO TASTE
1 TABLESPOON FRESH CHOPPED CHIVES

1. Put the mushrooms and water in a large container, and place in the refrigerator, covered, for about 8 hours.

2. When ready, drain off the mushroom water into another bowl or container. Press the mushrooms gently against the sieve to extract as much mushroom flavor as possible.

3. Stir the nama shoyu into the mushroom broth, and season with sea salt and black pepper to taste.

4. Remove and discard the stems from the mushrooms and chop the caps.

5. Add the chopped mushrooms to the broth and top with the chopped chives.

Spicy Tomato Soup

MAKES 4 SERVINGS

Tomatoes are best eaten like apples, fresh picked and still warm from the sun. Nothing compares to that fresh sweet taste, except perhaps this soup. Your tomatoes should be very ripe, and the sun-dried tomatoes softened enough to puree easily. Tomatoes, one of the healthiest fruits due to their high vitamin, beta carotene, and lycopene content, should be eaten every day to reduce the risk of several cancers.

8 LARGE RIPE TOMATOES, PEELED AND SEEDED

1 RED BELL PEPPER, SEEDED AND CHOPPED

1 SMALL JALAPEÑO PEPPER, SEEDED AND CHOPPED

1 MEDIUM ENGLISH CUCUMBER, PEELED AND CHOPPED

¾ CUP SUN-DRIED TOMATOES, SOAKED IN WATER
    TO SOFTEN AND DRAINED

3 TEASPOONS APPLE CIDER VINEGAR

¼ CUP FRESH CHOPPED BASIL

1 TEASPOON FRESH CHOPPED OREGANO

SEA SALT AND FRESHLY GROUND BLACK PEPPER

1. Place all the ingredients except the sea salt and black pepper in a blender, and process until very smooth.

2. Pour the soup through a sieve, pressing lightly, and season with the sea salt and black pepper to taste.

Cauliflower Apple Soup

Apple mellows out the cauliflower in this dish with a hint of sweetness and acid. The combination of these fiber-packed foods creates a soup that is delicious and a great detoxifier. To create the tastiest soup, use freshly grated nutmeg.

6 CUPS CHOPPED CAULIFLOWER FLORETS
2 LARGE TART APPLES, PEELED, CORED, AND CHOPPED
4 CUPS WATER
3 TABLESPOONS APPLE CIDER VINEGAR
3 TABLESPOONS EXTRA-VIRGIN OLIVE OIL
1 TABLESPOON AGAVE NECTAR
1 TEASPOON FRESHLY GRATED NUTMEG
SEA SALT AND FRESHLY GROUND BLACK PEPPER, TO TASTE
RAW SOUR CREAM (SEE RECIPE IN CHAPTER 12), TO GARNISH

1. Place all the ingredients except the salt, pepper, and raw sour cream in a blender, and process until smooth.

2. Pass the soup through a medium sieve, and season with the sea salt and black pepper to taste.

3. Top with the raw sour cream and serve chilled.

Cucumber Dill Soup

MAKES 4 SERVINGS

The best way to describe this soup is "spring in a bowl." Because the finished soup's texture is thin, let it sit a few minutes to allow the juices to purge and then season it. If you want a thicker soup, puree half an avocado with the rest of the ingredients. To add a satisfying crunch, try pureeing five cucumbers instead of six, and mince the remaining cucumber to stir in after the soup is prepared.

6 ENGLISH CUCUMBERS, PEELED AND ROUGHLY CHOPPED
JUICE AND ZEST OF 3 LEMONS
1 TEASPOON FRESH CHOPPED DILL
1 TEASPOON AGAVE NECTAR
½ TEASPOON MINCED GARLIC
SEA SALT AND FRESHLY GROUND BLACK PEPPER, TO TASTE
RAW SOUR CREAM (SEE RECIPE IN CHAPTER 12), FOR GARNISH

1. Place all the ingredients except the sea salt, black pepper, and garnish in a blender and process until smooth.

2. Season to taste and serve very cold with a dollop of sour cream.

Red Bell Pepper Soup

This deep-hued soup is sweet and fresh, and leaves just a hint of hotness on the tongue. Leave in a little of the red pepper pulp if you want a thicker soup, but the avocado actually bulks it up nicely without reducing the pure pepper taste. For an elegant presentation, consider adding a dash of raw sour cream along with the shreds of fresh basil.

16 RED BELL PEPPERS, SEEDED

2 RIPE AVOCADOS, PEELED, PITTED, AND PUREED

2 TABLESPOONS PURE MAPLE SYRUP

½ TEASPOON FINELY GRATED HORSERADISH

SEA SALT AND FRESHLY GROUND BLACK PEPPER, TO TASTE

FRESH BASIL, CUT INTO FINE CHIFFONADE, FOR GARNISH

1. Juice the red bell peppers and discard the pulp.

2. Measure out 6–7 cups of pepper juice into a large bowl.

3. Whisk the avocado, maple syrup, and horseradish into the juice until well combined.

4. Season with the sea salt and black pepper to taste.

5. Chill and garnish with basil.

Carrot Ginger Soup

MAKES 4–6 SERVINGS

Make this soup whenever you need a healthful pick-me-up up during cold-and-flu season. With its vibrant colors, this soup is chock-full of disease-fighting antioxidants from the carrots and ginger. Ginger, a natural health remedy used in many cultures, tastes best when freshly grated.

15 LARGE CARROTS, PEELED AND CHOPPED ROUGHLY

2 RIPE AVOCADOS, PEELED, PITTED, AND CHOPPED

½ CUP FRESHLY GRATED COCONUT

1 TABLESPOON MINCED GARLIC

1 TABLESPOON FRESHLY GRATED GINGER

JUICE OF 1 LEMON

SEA SALT AND FRESHLY GROUND BLACK PEPPER, TO TASTE

1. Juice the carrots in a juicer and discard the pulp.

2. Measure out 6 cups of carrot juice into a blender and add the remaining ingredients except the sea salt and black pepper, and process until smooth.

3. Season with the sea salt and black pepper to taste, and serve chilled.

Spicy Peanut Soup

MAKES 6 SERVINGS

In Western cultures, peanuts are mostly consumed as a quick snack or pureed into the incredibly popular spread found in almost every pantry. In North Africa, peanuts are a base ingredient in soups, sauces, and stews, such as this spicy and satisfying version. The flavor combinations might be a little unfamiliar at first, but you will soon find this the perfect dish for a hearty dinner accompanied by a fresh green salad.

8 CUPS FRESH CARROT JUICE

1 AVOCADO, PEELED AND PITTED

1 LARGE SWEET POTATO, PEELED AND DICED

½ JALAPEÑO PEPPER, SEEDED AND DICED

½ SMALL SWEET ONION, PEELED AND DICED

⅔ CUP RAW PEANUT BUTTER

5 TEASPOONS AGAVE NECTAR

JUICE AND ZEST OF 2 LIMES

1 TEASPOON FRESHLY GRATED GINGER

1 TEASPOON MINCED GARLIC

1 TEASPOON GROUND CUMIN

1 TEASPOON GROUND CINNAMON

MANGO CHUTNEY, FOR GARNISH

¼ CUP FRESH CHOPPED CILANTRO, FOR GARNISH

1. Place all the ingredients except the mango chutney and cilantro in a food processor and blend until smooth.

2. Transfer the soup to individual bowls, and serve with a spoonful of mango chutney and a sprinkling of cilantro.

Tortilla Soup

MAKES 4-6 SERVINGS

If you enjoy Mexican food, you will adore this colorful, complex soup. This is not a recipe you can whip together, however; it requires a bit of planning to create the crispy "tortilla" strips crucial to the end result. To save time, make a large batch of these tortilla strips ahead of time and store them in the refrigerator in a sealed container. If you like your food extra spicy, use a whole jalapeño pepper.

FOR THE SOUP:

6 LARGE RIPE TOMATOES, PEELED, SEEDED, AND CHOPPED

4 CELERY STALKS, CHOPPED

2 LARGE RED BELL PEPPERS, SEEDED AND CHOPPED

1 YELLOW BELL PEPPER, SEEDED AND CHOPPED

1 CUP WATER

⅔ CUP SUN-DRIED TOMATOES

½ CUP FRESH CHOPPED CILANTRO

JUICE AND ZEST OF 1 LIME

½ JALAPEÑO PEPPER, SEEDED AND CHOPPED

1 TEASPOON MINCED GARLIC

1 TEASPOON GROUND CUMIN

½ TEASPOON GROUND CORIANDER

½ TEASPOON CHILI POWDER

PINCH OF CAYENNE PEPPER

SEA SALT AND FRESHLY GROUND BLACK PEPPER, TO TASTE

¼ CUP EXTRA-VIRGIN OLIVE OIL

GUACAMOLE, FOR GARNISH

FOR THE "TORTILLA" STRIPS:

1 EZEKIEL WRAP

Make the soup:

1. Place all the ingredients except the olive oil and garnish in a food processor, and pulse until well combined but a little chunky.

2. While the processor is still running, add the olive oil in a thin stream until the soup is emulsified.

3. Adjust the seasonings.

Make the "tortilla" strips:

1. Cut the Ezekiel wrap into strips.

2. Crisp the strips in an oven at very low heat.

3. Serve the soup topped with guacamole and "tortilla" strips.

CHAPTER NINE

Salads

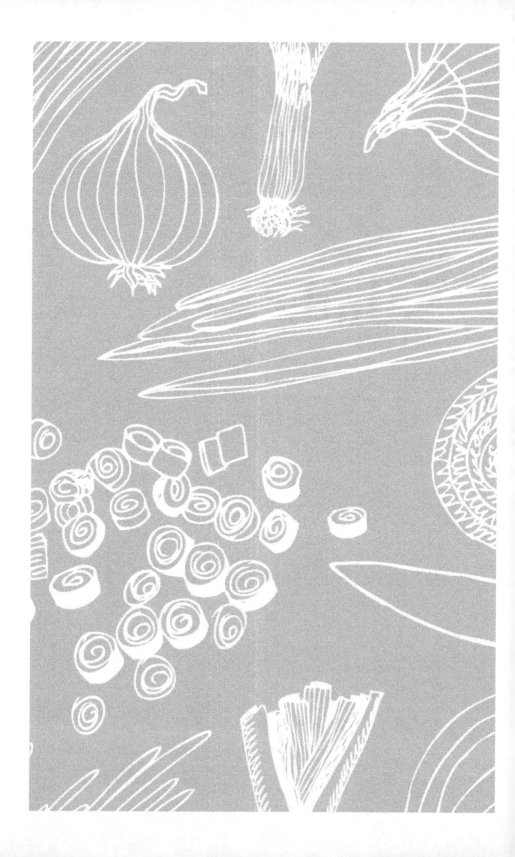

Curried Cabbage Slaw

MAKES 6 SERVINGS

A satisfying meal in itself, this salad is best when you make it ahead of time and allow all the flavors to mellow. You can substitute dried cranberries for the raisins in this dish and add sunflower or pumpkin seeds for even more crunch and texture.

1 HEAD NAPA CABBAGE, SHREDDED

½ HEAD RED CABBAGE, SHREDDED

3 LARGE CARROTS, PEELED AND SHREDDED

½ RED ONION, SLICED VERY THIN

1 CUP UNSWEETENED SHREDDED COCONUT

½ CUP RAISINS

SEA SALT, TO TASTE

½ CUP RAW SOUR CREAM (SEE RECIPE IN CHAPTER 12)

¼ CUP SESAME SEEDS

2 TABLESPOONS FRESH LEMON JUICE

1 TABLESPOON AGAVE NECTAR

1 TABLESPOON NAMA SHOYU

1 TEASPOON GROUND CUMIN

½ TEASPOON CURRY POWDER

¼ TEASPOON GROUND TURMERIC

1. Place the cabbages, carrots, red onion, shredded coconut, and raisins in a large bowl, and toss to combine well. Season with the sea salt to taste.

2. Add the raw sour cream, sesame seeds, lemon juice, agave nectar, nama shoyu, cumin, curry powder, and turmeric to the cabbage mixture, and toss to combine.

3. Place slaw in the refrigerator for at least 2 hours to let the flavors mellow.

Waldorf Salad

Waldorf salad made its first appearance in 1893 in New York City at the hands of the maître d'hôtel of the Waldorf Astoria, Oscar Tschirky. Originally the salad was a tasty mix of celery, apples, and mayonnaise. Chopped pecans and grapes followed afterward. This raw version is even more delicious with the addition of tangy yogurt and a hint of mint and sweetness. Enjoy it as a main course whenever you want a light, refreshing meal.

2 GREEN APPLES, CORED AND DICED

2 CUPS RED SEEDLESS GRAPES, HALVED

4 STALKS CELERY, FINELY DICED

1½ CUPS CHOPPED PECANS

1 TABLESPOON FRESH CHOPPED MINT

1 TABLESPOON PURE MAPLE SYRUP

½ TEASPOON FRESH LEMON JUICE

½ CUP RAW YOGURT

4 CUPS WATERCRESS, OPTIONAL

1. In a large bowl toss together the apples, grapes, celery, and pecans until well mixed.

2. In a small bowl stir together the mint, maple syrup, lemon juice, and yogurt until well blended.

3. Add the dressing to the salad and toss to coat.

4. Serve chilled spooned onto watercress, if desired, or plain.

Avocado Mango Broccoli Salad

MAKES 2 SERVINGS

This tart salad is crunchy and very filling. When you toss the ingredients together, the avocado, if very ripe, creates a creamy dressing. Use firmer fruit if you don't want this effect.

3 LARGE RIPE MANGOES, PEELED, PITTED, AND CUT INTO STRIPS
2 LARGE RIPE AVOCADOS, PEELED, PITTED, AND CUBED
1 HEAD BROCCOLI, CHOPPED INTO BITE-SIZED FLORETS
1 CUP DRIED CRANBERRIES
½ CUP PUMPKIN SEEDS
SEA SALT AND FRESHLY GROUND BLACK PEPPER, TO TASTE

1. In a large bowl toss together all the ingredients until well combined.

2. Chill and serve.

Jicama and Melon Salad with Coriander-Cucumber Dressing

Jicama is one of those spectacular ingredients that is underused due to unfamiliarity. A rather ugly member of the potato family, it hides a surprisingly moist crispness under its unassuming thin brown skin, which makes it perfect in salads. Jicama is also very healthful, with almost no fat, few calories, and little sodium. It is also an excellent source of calcium, vitamin C, fiber, potassium, and iron.

FOR THE DRESSING:

½ CUP ALMONDS, SOAKED IN WATER FOR 4 HOURS,
    RINSED, AND DRAINED

1 MEDIUM ENGLISH CUCUMBER, PEELED AND SLICED

1 CLOVE GARLIC

1 TABLESPOON AGAVE NECTAR

JUICE OF 1 LIME

1 TEASPOON GROUND CORIANDER

½ TEASPOON GROUND CUMIN

SEA SALT AND FRESHLY GROUND BLACK PEPPER, TO TASTE

FOR THE SALAD:

4 CUPS JICAMA, PEELED AND CUT INTO THIN STRIPS

4 CUPS CANTALOUPE, CUBED

2 CUPS CHERRY TOMATOES, HALVED

1 CUP PUMPKIN SEEDS

3 SCALLIONS, THINLY SLICED

Make the dressing:

1. Place all the dressing ingredients except the sea salt and black pepper in a blender, and pulse until smooth. Season with the sea salt and black pepper to taste.

Make the salad:

1. Place the salad ingredients in a large bowl and toss to combine.

2. Toss the salad with the dressing and serve chilled.

Kale Broccoli Salad

MAKES 4 SERVINGS

With its deep purple, dark green, and vibrant red ingredients dappled with orange zest and jewel-like cranberries, this salad should be presented proudly to guests on your heirloom serving platter. The sweet maple dressing is an especially nice surprise. For a real treat, try adding ripe plump blackberries if they are in season.

FOR THE DRESSING:

JUICE AND ZEST OF 1 ORANGE

1 TABLESPOON PURE MAPLE SYRUP

1 TABLESPOON BALSAMIC VINEGAR

SEA SALT AND FRESHLY GROUND BLACK PEPPER, TO TASTE

¼ CUP EXTRA-VIRGIN OLIVE OIL

FOR THE SALAD:

6 CUPS PURPLE KALE, SHREDDED

2 CUPS SMALL BROCCOLI FLORETS, CHOPPED ROUGHLY

2 CUPS HALVED CHERRY TOMATOES

2 SCALLIONS, THINLY SLICED

1 CUP DRIED CRANBERRIES

¼ CUP PUMPKIN SEEDS, FOR GARNISH

Make the dressing:

1. Combine the orange juice, zest, maple syrup, and balsamic vinegar in a blender, and pulse until mixed.

2. Season with the sea salt and black pepper to taste.

3. While the blender is running, add the olive oil in a thin stream until the dressing emulsifies.

Make the salad:

1. Toss all the salad ingredients except the pumpkin seeds in a large bowl.

2. Toss the salad with the dressing until well coated.

3. Top with the pumpkin seeds and serve.

Primavera Pesto Salad

In this kitchen-sink approach to salad making, you can substitute almost any vegetable here and get a good result. For example, you can use carrot ribbons instead of sprouts and add some cherry tomatoes for a change of pace. Experiment and discover new favorite combinations to satisfy your palate.

4–5 CUPS MIXED SPROUTS
2 CUPS SHREDDED BABY SPINACH
½ CUP FRESH BASIL OR HERB PESTO
6 BEETS, PEELED AND SLIVERED
1 CUP SMALL CAULIFLOWER FLORETS
2 SMALL CARROTS, PEELED AND SLICED INTO
   VERY THIN STRIPS
1 BUNCH WATERCRESS

1. Toss the sprouts and spinach with the pesto in a large bowl until well coated.

2. Add the remaining ingredients and toss to combine.

Spinach Mango Salad

MAKES 2 LARGE SERVINGS

Many newbies to the raw diet find themselves eating a great deal of salads because salads are familiar and simple to make. This salad is a perfect starter or main course for raw food enthusiasts. The ingredients are easy to find, and no special techniques are required to prepare it. The dressing is a traditional balsamic vinaigrette and can be used with other salads, so make extra and store it in a bottle in your refrigerator.

FOR THE DRESSING:

2 TABLESPOONS BALSAMIC VINEGAR

1 TABLESPOON AGAVE NECTAR

1 TEASPOON FRESH CHOPPED THYME

¼ CUP EXTRA-VIRGIN OLIVE OIL

SEA SALT AND FRESHLY GROUND BLACK PEPPER, TO TASTE

FOR THE SALAD:

4 CUPS BABY SPINACH

2 CUPS ARUGULA

2 LARGE MANGOS, PEELED, PITTED, AND SLICED

2 SMALL ENGLISH CUCUMBERS, DICED

½ CUP PISTACHIOS, CHOPPED

Make the dressing:

1. Whisk together the balsamic vinegar, agave nectar, and thyme in a small bowl until well blended.

2. Add the olive oil in a thin stream, whisking until emulsified. Season with the sea salt and black pepper to taste.

Make the salad:

1. Toss the salad ingredients together except the pistachios until well mixed.

2. Toss the salad with the dressing and serve topped with chopped pistachios.

Watermelon Lime Salad

MAKES 4-6 SERVINGS

Watermelon, synonymous with hot summer days, makes this salad a welcome addition to any meal or gathering. The tart lime dressing enhances the sweetness of the melon and peaches while playing up the crispness of the jicama. You can use yellow or red watermelon in this recipe or mix them together for an interesting contrast.

FOR THE DRESSING:

JUICE AND ZEST OF 2 LIMES

2 TABLESPOONS RAW HONEY

1 TABLESPOON APPLE CIDER VINEGAR

¼ CUP EXTRA-VIRGIN OLIVE OIL

SEA SALT AND FRESHLY GROUND BLACK PEPPER, TO TASTE

FOR THE SALAD:

1 SEEDLESS WATERMELON, PEELED AND DICED

1 JICAMA, PEELED AND DICED

6 RIPE PEACHES, PITTED AND THINLY SLICED

1 SCALLION, THINLY SLICED

½ CUP SUNFLOWER SEEDS

Make the dressing:

1. Whisk together all the dressing ingredients except the olive oil and the sea salt and black pepper. Add the olive oil in a thin stream until the dressing emulsifies.

2. Season with the sea salt and black pepper to taste.

Make the salad:

1. Toss the watermelon, jicama, peaches, and scallion together in a large bowl until well combined.

2. Toss the salad with the dressing and top with sunflower seeds.

Asian Pear Jicama Salad

Crisp and juicy, tart and sweet, this salad requires a bit of prep time, but the end result is well worth the effort. Precise cutting creates the delicate, rich appearance of the salad and will ensure that each bite has the perfect combination of flavors and textures. This salad is best eaten right away. If left too long, the Asian pear will oxidize into an unpleasant brownish color.

3 ASIAN PEARS, CORED AND DICED

1 JICAMA, PEELED AND DICED

2 SMALL CARROTS, PEELED AND JULIENNED

1 SMALL ENGLISH CUCUMBER, DICED

JUICE AND ZEST OF 1 LIME

½ CUP DRIED CRANBERRIES

3 TABLESPOONS EXTRA-VIRGIN OLIVE OIL

2 TABLESPOONS FRESH CHOPPED MINT

1 TABLESPOON FRESH CHOPPED PARSLEY

SEA SALT AND FRESHLY GROUND BLACK PEPPER, TO TASTE

1. Toss all the ingredients except the sea salt and black pepper in a large bowl.

2. Season with the sea salt and black pepper to taste.

Avocado and Beet Greens Salad

If you are looking for a robust salad, search no further. This is a salad to tote in a huge picnic basket because it will take some jostling with no ill effects. The segmented oranges in this recipe don't need to look perfect, because their appearance isn't important to the finished dish. Simply follow the membranes on the orange as closely as possible and take your time.

FOR THE DRESSING:

2 NAVEL ORANGES

¼ CUP FRESH ORANGE JUICE, FROM CUTTING THE ORANGES

½ TEASPOON FRESHLY GRATED ORANGE ZEST

2 TABLESPOONS APPLE CIDER VINEGAR

2 TABLESPOONS AGAVE NECTAR

1 TEASPOON FRESHLY GRATED GINGER

¼ CUP EXTRA-VIRGIN OLIVE OIL

SEA SALT AND FRESHLY GROUND BLACK PEPPER, TO TASTE

FOR THE SALAD:

6 CUPS BABY BEET GREENS

SEGMENTS FROM 2 NAVEL ORANGES, RESERVED FROM DRESSING

1 RIPE AVOCADO, PEELED, PITTED, AND DICED

1 CUP PUMPKIN SEEDS

Make the dressing:

1. Cut the skin off the oranges with a very sharp paring knife until just the flesh remains.

2. Take the knife and cut each segment out of the orange, using the membranes as a guide and making sure you cut over a bowl to catch the juice.

3. Set the segments aside to use in the salad.

continued ▶

4. In a small bowl whisk together all the dressing ingredients except the olive oil, sea salt, and black pepper until well blended.

5. Whisk in the olive oil in a thin stream until the dressing emulsifies, and season with the sea salt and black pepper to taste.

Make the salad:

1. Dress the beet greens with the dressing.

2. Top with the reserved orange segments, avocado, and pumpkin seeds.

CHAPTER TEN

Entrées

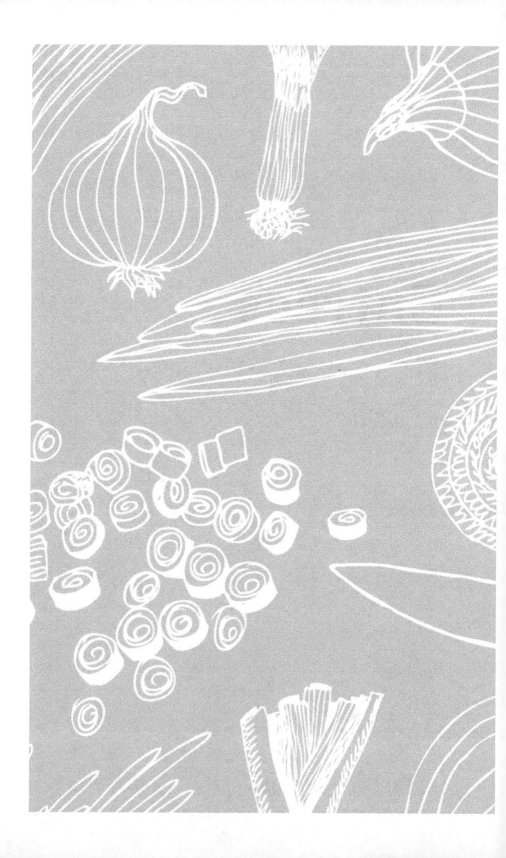

Coconut Pad Thai

MAKES 4 LARGE SERVINGS

With its incredible depth of flavor, pad thai has become immensely popular recently. This raw version obviously doesn't use noodles, but you'll be surprised by how much the coconut strands mimic their processed counterparts. Pad thai is best when you allow it to sit in the refrigerator at least a few hours to mellow the flavors.

FOR THE SAUCE:

3 TABLESPOONS RAW PEANUT BUTTER

2 TABLESPOONS PURE MAPLE SYRUP

2 TABLESPOONS NAMA SHOYU

2 TABLESPOONS MINCED GARLIC

1 TABLESPOON EXTRA-VIRGIN OLIVE OIL

1 TEASPOON MINCED CHILI PEPPER

DASH OF SEA SALT

FOR THE VEGETABLES:

2 CUPS SHREDDED NAPA CABBAGE

2 CUPS FRESH JULIENNED COCONUT

2 CUPS SHREDDED CARROT

1 CUP JULIENNED GREEN ZUCCHINI

½ SMALL SWEET ONION, VERY THINLY SLICED

2 SCALLIONS, THINLY SLICED

1 HOT CHILI PEPPER, VERY THINLY SLICED

½ CUP FRESH CHOPPED CILANTRO

3 TABLESPOONS CHOPPED PEANUTS

Make the sauce:

1. In a medium bowl whisk together all the sauce ingredients until well combined. Set aside.

continued ▶

Coconut Pad Thai *continued* ▶

Make the vegetables:

1. In a large bowl toss together all the ingredients except the cilantro and chopped peanuts until well mixed.

2. Add the sauce to the vegetables and toss to combine.

3. Serve topped with the cilantro and peanuts.

Pasta with Pistachio Pesto

MAKES 4 SERVINGS

Most commercial pesto is made with pine nuts and basil, but substituting other nuts can create tasty variations that work just as well. Pistachios are perfect for pesto. Their mild, sweet taste plays up the basil, allowing the herb to shine. This dish is as close to actual pasta as the raw diet gets because kelp noodles have a similar texture to "real" noodles. Read your labels carefully when purchasing kelp noodles. Some are not raw, due to production methods.

10 CUPS RAW KELP NOODLES, WITH ENOUGH
   WARM WATER TO COVER
2 CUPS PACKED FRESH BASIL LEAVES
1 CUP PISTACHIOS
½ CUP EXTRA-VIRGIN OLIVE OIL
1 LARGE GARLIC CLOVE
SEA SALT AND FRESHLY GROUND BLACK PEPPER, TO TASTE
2 CUPS SMALL BROCCOLI FLORETS
2 CUPS HALVED CHERRY TOMATOES

1. Place the kelp noodles in a large bowl and cover with warm water. Soak for about 30 minutes.

2. To make the pesto, place the basil leaves, pistachios, olive oil, and garlic in a blender and process until smooth but still textured. Season with the sea salt and black pepper to taste.

3. Drain and rinse the kelp noodles and return to the bowl.

4. Add the broccoli and tomatoes, and toss to combine.

5. Add enough pesto to suit your taste, and toss to coat the noodles and vegetables.

Mixed Vegetable Curry with Parsnip Nut Rice

Although this dish takes a bit of time to prepare, it is spectacular and a good choice when serving people who don't follow a raw diet. The parsnip nut rice can be made a day in advance and stored in the refrigerator until you need to use it. Don't use raw wild parsnips because they can be toxic.

FOR THE VEGETABLES:

2 ½ CUPS PEELED AND DICED EGGPLANT

2 CUPS DICED PORTOBELLO MUSHROOMS

1 CUP BROCCOLI FLORETS

1 CUP FRESH SHELLED PEAS

8 MEDIUM TOMATOES, SEEDED AND DICED SMALL

2 TABLESPOONS CURRY POWDER

2 TABLESPOONS TAMARI

2 TABLESPOONS EXTRA-VIRGIN OLIVE OIL

2 TEASPOONS FRESH LEMON JUICE

1 TEASPOON SEA SALT

FOR THE CURRY SAUCE:

1 RED BELL PEPPER, SEEDED AND CHOPPED

¾ CUP FRESHLY GRATED COCONUT MEAT

½ CUP FRESH CHOPPED CILANTRO

⅓ CUP WATER

1 CLOVE GARLIC, ROUGHLY CHOPPED

1 TABLESPOON CURRY POWDER

1 TEASPOON GROUND CUMIN

1 TEASPOON FRESH LEMON JUICE

¼-INCH PIECE FRESH GINGER, PEELED

SEA SALT, TO TASTE

FOR THE PARSNIP NUT RICE:

4 LARGE PARSNIPS, PEELED AND CHOPPED INTO CHUNKS

¼ CUP PINE NUTS

¼ CUP ALMONDS

1 TABLESPOON AGAVE NECTAR

2 TEASPOONS EXTRA-VIRGIN OLIVE OIL

2 TEASPOONS WHITE MISO

1 TEASPOON FRESH LEMON JUICE

SEA SALT, TO TASTE

Make the vegetables:

1. In a large bowl toss all the ingredients together until well mixed.

2. Transfer the vegetables to two dehydrator sheets, and dehydrate them for about 3 hours at 105 degrees F.

Make the curry sauce:

1. Transfer all the ingredients to a blender, and pulse until smooth.

2. Adjust the seasonings.

3. Add the curry sauce to the dehydrated vegetables in a serving bowl, and toss to combine.

For the parsnip nut rice:

1. Place all the ingredients except the sea salt in a food processor, and pulse until it has a rice consistency.

2. Season with the sea salt to taste.

3. Serve the curry over the rice.

Falafel

MAKES 4 SERVINGS

Falafel, a popular vegetarian dish, is usually deep-fried. This raw version can be served wrapped in a raw tortilla or on its own with a creamy sauce or simple marinara. You can substitute green olives for black ones in this recipe. If you do, remember to use a little less salt to offset the different tastes.

2 CUPS PUMPKIN SEEDS

½ CUP PITTED KALAMATA OLIVES

½ CUP SUN-DRIED TOMATO HALVES, SOAKED IN
    WATER TO SOFTEN AND CHOPPED

⅓ CUP FRESH CHOPPED CILANTRO

¼ CUP FRESH DILL LEAVES, FINELY CHOPPED

4 MEDIUM SHALLOTS

2 CLOVES GARLIC

2 TABLESPOONS GROUND CUMIN

2 TABLESPOONS DRIED OREGANO

2 TABLESPOONS FRESH LEMON JUICE

1 TABLESPOON GROUND CORIANDER

½ TEASPOON SEA SALT

PINCH OF CAYENNE PEPPER

PINCH OF FRESHLY GROUND BLACK PEPPER

RAW TORTILLAS (SEE RECIPE IN CHAPTER 12)
    OR RAW TZATZIKI SAUCE, FOR SERVING

1. Place all the ingredients in a food processor, and pulse until the mixture holds together.

2. Form mixture into balls about the size of golf balls, and place on dehydrator sheets.

3. Dehydrate for 7–8 hours at 105 degrees F.

4. Serve wrapped in a raw tortilla or with raw tzatziki sauce.

Mushroom Nut Sausage

MAKES 4 SERVINGS

Portobello mushrooms are often used as a meat substitute in vegetarian cuisine. In this dish their texture creates real substance and provides a wonderful base for the rest of the ingredients. Add this sausage to tomato sauces, chili, and ratatouille-style dishes to create healthful variations. This dish uses zucchini noodles, which can be created by either cutting thin strips or using a tool called a spiralizer. The initial stage in the dehydrator uses a higher temperature than what is usually recommended for raw food, but since the sausage never reaches that temperature, it is okay.

3 CUPS FINELY CHOPPED PORTOBELLO MUSHROOMS

3 CUPS GRATED CARROTS

1½ CUPS SWEET ONION, PEELED AND FINELY CHOPPED

1¼ CUPS DICED CELERY

1⅓ CUPS PECANS, SOAKED IN WATER FOR 4–6 HOURS
    AND GROUND FINE WHILE WET

⅔ CUP PUMPKIN SEEDS, SOAKED IN WATER FOR 8 HOURS
    AND GROUND FINE WHILE WET

⅓ CUP WATER

⅓ CUP NAMA SHOYU

1 TEASPOON DRIED OREGANO

1 TEASPOON DRIED BASIL

½ TEASPOON DRIED THYME

1¼ CUP GROUND FLAXSEED

ZUCCHINI PASTA OR "ROASTED" VEGETABLE SAUCE,
    FOR SERVING

1. In a large bowl stir together the mushrooms, carrots, onion, and celery until well mixed.

2. Add the pecans and pumpkin seeds, and combine well.

continued ▶

3. In a small bowl stir together the water and nama shoyu, and stir it into the mushroom mixture.

4. Stir in the dried herbs and add the ground flaxseed in two batches, mixing until well combined.

5. Shape the mixture into patties about 1 inch thick and 5 inches in diameter.

6. Place the patties onto dehydrator screens, and dehydrate for about 1 hour at 140 degrees F. Reduce the heat to 105 degrees F, and dehydrate for about 8 hours until completely dry.

7. Cut into bite-sized pieces and serve with zucchini pasta or in a "roasted" vegetable sauce.

Mediterranean "Roasted" Vegetables

MAKES 3 SERVINGS

Since grilled vegetables aren't allowed on a raw diet, this dish is a tasty substitute. The combinations of vegetables and amounts used can be changed to reflect your personal taste. You can also add sun-dried tomatoes for a meatier texture.

½ SMALL EGGPLANT, DICED

1 SMALL GREEN ZUCCHINI, SLICED

1 SMALL YELLOW ZUCCHINI, SLICED

1 RED BELL PEPPER, SEEDED AND DICED

1 MEDIUM RED ONION, SLICED INTO ROUNDS

1 LARGE TOMATO, SLICED

¼ CUP EXTRA-VIRGIN OLIVE OIL

2 TABLESPOONS FRESH LEMON JUICE

½ TEASPOON SEA SALT

FRESHLY GROUND BLACK PEPPER, TO TASTE

1. In a large bowl toss together all the ingredients, and let sit in the refrigerator for at least 2–3 hours to marinate.

2. Transfer the vegetables to dehydrator sheets, and place in dehydrator for about 2 hours at 105 degrees F, or until softened.

3. Adjust the seasonings.

Simple Marinara Sauce

Keep a jar of this rich tomato sauce on hand. It's perfect for a main-course meal, dip, and even as a spread for raw sandwiches. Place the noodles in a strainer to drain for about thirty minutes before using them. Otherwise their liquid could make your sauce watery.

4 CUPS SUN-DRIED TOMATOES, SOAKED IN WATER
    UNTIL VERY SOFT, AND DRAINED
3 CLOVES GARLIC
1 TABLESPOON DRIED BASIL
1 TABLESPOON DRIED OREGANO
SEA SALT AND FRESHLY GROUND BLACK PEPPER, TO TASTE
4 FIRM ZUCCHINI, PUT THROUGH A SPIRALIZER
    OR CUT INTO LONG THIN STRIPS

1. Place all of the ingredients except the zucchini in a blender and process until smooth. Leave a little texture if you like your sauce chunkier.

2. Adjust the seasonings and serve over zucchini noodles.

Vegetable Chili

MAKES 4 LARGE SERVINGS

People take their chili seriously. Like its meat-based counterpart, this raw version tastes best at least four hours after cooking, which allows the spices and flavors to blend. Use this dish as a main course topped with raw sour cream and nut cheeses, or as a dip.

6 LARGE RIPE TOMATOES, PEELED, SEEDED, AND DICED

2 CUPS HALVED GRAPE TOMATOES

2 GREEN BELL PEPPERS, SEEDED AND DICED

2 JALAPEÑO PEPPERS, SEEDED AND MINCED

1 CUP SUNFLOWER SEEDS

1 LARGE CARROT, PEELED AND GRATED

1 TEASPOON MINCED GARLIC

1 TEASPOON CHILI POWDER

1 TEASPOON GROUND CUMIN

¼ CUP RAW SOUR CREAM (SEE RECIPE IN CHAPTER 12)

1. Place all the ingredients except the sour cream in a large bowl, and toss to combine well.

2. Serve topped with the raw sour cream or use as a dip.

Vegetable Sarma

MAKES 6 SERVINGS

Dolmas are a stuffed vegetable dish popular in the Balkans. When the filling is placed in grape or cabbage leaves, the dish is called "sarma." Finding brined grape leaves can be difficult, but most Middle Eastern markets will have them in jars or cans. If you cannot find these leaves, use this tasty filling in tomatoes or peppers.

1 SMALL CAULIFLOWER HEAD, CHOPPED
    AND PROCESSED TO LOOK LIKE RICE
½ CUP MINCED SWEET ONION, DEHYDRATED FOR
    20 MINUTES AT 115 DEGREES F
2 STALKS CELERY, CHOPPED
½ CUP PINE NUTS
1 LARGE CLOVE GARLIC
3 TABLESPOONS FRESH LEMON JUICE, DIVIDED
½ CUP FRESH MINCED PARSLEY
⅓ CUP RAISINS, SOAKED IN WATER FOR 1 HOUR AND DRAINED
¼ CUP FRESH CHOPPED MINT
ZEST OF 1 LEMON
SEA SALT, TO TASTE
2 TABLESPOONS EXTRA-VIRGIN OLIVE OIL
12 BRINED GRAPE LEAVES

1. Place the cauliflower and onion in a large bowl.

2. Place the celery, pine nuts, garlic clove, and 2 tablespoons lemon juice in a blender, and process until well combined.

3. Add the celery mixture to the cauliflower along with the parsley, raisins, mint, lemon zest, and sea salt, and stir to combine.

4. Mix together the olive oil and the remaining 1 tablespoon lemon juice in a small bowl.

5. Place 1 grape leaf stem side down on a work surface, and brush it with the olive oil mixture.

6. Spoon about 4 tablespoons of the filling at the base of the leaf, and roll it up like a cigar, tucking in the edges as you roll.

7. Brush a little more of the olive oil mixture on the rolled leaf, and set it aside on a plate seam side down.

8. Repeat the process with the remaining grape leaves.

Stuffed Peppers

This wonderfully filling meal is very close to the traditional meat-filled version. You can even top these with shredded nut cheese. The nuts in this filling can be replaced with other types, such as macadamia and cashews, if desired.

1⅓ CUPS PECANS, SOAKED IN WATER FOR 10 HOURS, RINSED, AND DRAINED

1⅓ CUPS PINE NUTS, SOAKED IN WATER FOR 6 HOURS, RINSED, AND DRAINED

2 TOMATOES, SEEDED AND DICED

⅔ CUP FRESH CORN KERNELS

1 SCALLION, FINELY SLICED

½ CUP FRESH CHOPPED CILANTRO

3 TEASPOONS RAW MISO

3 TEASPOONS EXTRA-VIRGIN OLIVE OIL

1 TABLESPOON FRESHLY GRATED GINGER

1 TABLESPOON FRESH LEMON JUICE

1 TABLESPOON MINCED GARLIC

1 TEASPOON GROUND CORIANDER

1 TEASPOON GROUND CUMIN

1 TEASPOON FRESH MINCED OREGANO

½ TEASPOON CHILI POWDER

8 SMALL GREEN PEPPERS, SEEDED AND STEMMED

1. Place the pecans and pine nuts in a food processor, and pulse until well blended.

2. Add the remaining ingredients except the green peppers, and pulse until combined.

3. Spoon the pecan mixture into the green peppers, filling them evenly.

4. Place the stuffed green peppers on a nonstick sheet.

5. Dehydrate the green peppers for 8 hours at 115 degrees F until tender but still firm.

CHAPTER ELEVEN

Desserts

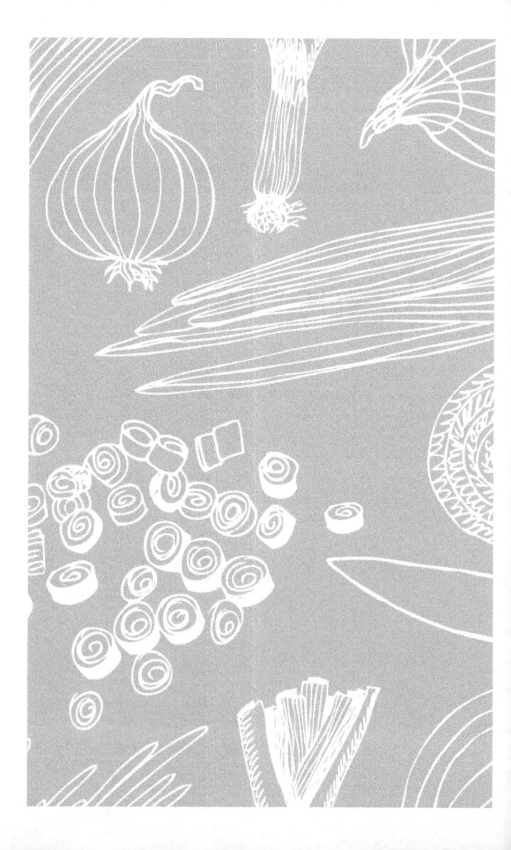

Chocolate Brownies

MAKES 16 BROWNIES

Serve this dessert to people who say they don't like raw food. Topped with a creamy raw vanilla bean ice cream, it will convert anyone to this style of eating. For neat portions, let these treats set up completely in the freezer before cutting them.

1 CUP ALMONDS, SOAKED IN WATER FOR 6 HOURS,
    RINSED, AND DRAINED
½ CUP CASHEWS, SOAKED IN WATER FOR 6 HOURS,
    RINSED, AND DRAINED
1½ CUPS PITTED DATES
⅔ CUP COCOA POWDER

1. Line an 8 × 8–inch baking dish with parchment paper and set aside.

2. Place all the ingredients in a food processor, and process until the mixture resembles cookie crumbs.

3. Spoon the mixture into the prepared pan, and press down firmly.

4. Place the pan in the freezer until the brownies are set, about 2 hours.

5. Take the pan out of the freezer, and flip it upside down onto a cutting board.

6. Peel off the parchment paper, and cut into 16 equal squares.

7. Store the brownies in the freezer in an airtight container.

Fresh Strawberry Pie

A good source of antioxidants and phytonutrients, strawberries taste best in season so try to make this pie at their peak of flavor and freshness. You can substitute other fruits such as berries and peaches when strawberry season is over.

FOR THE CRUST:

1 TABLESPOON COCONUT OIL, PLUS MORE
    TO GREASE PIE PLATE

2 CUPS ALMONDS

SEEDS FROM ½ VANILLA BEAN, SCRAPED OUT

PINCH OF SEA SALT

6 MEDJOOL DATES, PITTED

FOR THE FILLING:

2 CUPS CASHEWS, SOAKED IN WATER FOR 2-4 HOURS,
    RINSED, AND DRAINED

1 CUP SLICED STRAWBERRIES

¾ CUP MELTED COCONUT OIL

⅓ CUP AGAVE NECTAR

¼ CUP WATER

¼ CUP FRESH LEMON JUICE

1 TABLESPOON PURE VANILLA EXTRACT

¼ TEASPOON SEA SALT

FOR THE TOPPING:

2-3 CUPS SLICED STRAWBERRIES, DIVIDED

Make the crust:

1. Lightly oil a pie plate and set aside.

2. Transfer the almonds to a food processor, and pulse until they resemble coarse crumbs.

3. Add coconut oil, vanilla seeds, and sea salt, and pulse until combined.

4. Add the dates to the processor, and pulse until the crust starts to hold together. If the crust is too crumbly, add another date.

5. Press the crust into the prepared pie plate.

6. Chill the crust in the freezer for 30–60 minutes before adding the filling.

Make the filling:

1. Place all the filling ingredients in a blender, and pulse until the filling is smooth and thick.

2. Spoon half of the filling into the chilled pie shell; then place half of the sliced strawberries evenly over the filling.

3. Spoon the rest of the filling into the shell, and chill in the freezer for about 2 hours.

4. Top with the remaining sliced strawberries.

5. Serve cold.

Orange Chia Pudding

Complete a relaxed family meal with this comforting pudding. The oranges should be juicy, and be sure to wash the skin well before zesting it to remove any pesticides. For special occasions, top this pudding with a spoonful of vanilla cream. It will taste a lot like a Creamsicle.

½ CUP ALMONDS, SOAKED OVERNIGHT IN WATER,
    RINSED, AND DRAINED
2 CUPS WATER
6 DATES, PITTED
ZEST OF 2 ORANGES
6 LARGE ORANGES, DIVIDED
⅔ CUP CHIA SEEDS

1. Process the almonds and water in a blender until smooth.

2. Transfer the almond mixture to a piece of cheesecloth, and squeeze the liquid out into the blender. Discard the almonds or reserve them for another recipe.

3. Add the dates to the almond milk in the blender, and puree until smooth.

4. Transfer the date mixture to a large bowl, and add the orange zest.

5. Peel 2 of the oranges, and separate them into segments. Cut the segments in half. Set aside.

6. Juice the remaining 4 oranges, and add about 1½ cups juice to the date mixture and stir.

7. Add the chia seeds to the bowl and stir.

8. Let the mixture sit for about 30 minutes.

9. Stir in the orange sections and serve.

Banana Parfaits with Spiced Caramel Topping

MAKES 4 SERVINGS

This show-stopper of a dessert has many parts, so be sure you follow the recipe closely. For best results, the bananas should be very ripe. It's worth waiting until the skins get a few brown spots before making the dish.

FOR THE PARFAIT CRUMBLE:

1 CUP CHOPPED PECANS

2 TABLESPOONS AGAVE NECTAR

1 TABLESPOON COCONUT BUTTER

¼ TEASPOON GROUND NUTMEG

¼ TEASPOON GROUND ALLSPICE

¼ TEASPOON GROUND CINNAMON

FOR THE CARAMEL:

¾ CUP PURE MAPLE SYRUP

½ CUP COCONUT BUTTER, SOFTENED

¼ TEASPOON GROUND NUTMEG

¼ TEASPOON GROUND ALLSPICE

1 TEASPOON PURE VANILLA EXTRACT

PINCH OF SEA SALT

FOR THE BANANA FILLING:

1½ CUPS ALMONDS, SOAKED IN WATER FOR 8–12 HOURS
    UNTIL SOFT, RINSED, AND DRAINED

1 CUP FRESH COCONUT MEAT, CHOPPED

½ CUP COCONUT BUTTER, SOFTENED

⅓ CUP AGAVE NECTAR

¼ CUP COCONUT WATER

1 TEASPOON PURE VANILLA EXTRACT

4 LARGE RIPE BANANAS, PEELED, SLICED, TOSSED WITH
    2 TABLESPOONS FRESH LEMON JUICE, AND DRAINED

continued ▶

Make the parfait crumble:

1. Put all the ingredients in a food processor, and pulse until the mixture resembles coarse crumbs. Set aside in a bowl.

Make the caramel:

1. In a medium bowl combine all the ingredients, and whisk until smooth.

2. Put aside in a warm place so the sauce doesn't harden before you use it.

Make the banana filling:

1. Place all the ingredients except the bananas in a blender and process until smooth.

2. Transfer the filling to a bowl.

3. Mix the banana slices into the filling, and stir to combine.

4. Take 4 large glasses, and first place a layer of crumble in the bottom of each. Next add about 2 tablespoons of caramel sauce.

5. Add a thick layer of filling, and then repeat all three layers.

6. Top the second banana filling layer with crumble and a drizzle of caramel.

Dark Chocolate Gelato

MAKES 4 CUPS

Less thick and creamy than regular ice cream, this gelato still packs a rich chocolaty taste with a hint of sweet almond. Dark chocolate is loaded with antioxidants as well as many minerals, which can help promote a healthy cardiovascular system and help regulate blood sugar. Serve this treat with fresh berries and chopped crunchy nuts, if desired.

3 CUPS ALMOND MILK (SEE RECIPE IN CHAPTER 12)

1½ CUPS FRESH CHOPPED COCONUT MEAT

1½ CUPS UNSWEETENED COCONUT MILK

⅔ CUP AGAVE NECTAR

¾ CUP COCOA POWDER

3 TABLESPOONS COCONUT OIL

SEEDS FROM 1 VANILLA BEAN, SCRAPED OUT

1. Place all the ingredients in a blender, and process until smooth.

2. Transfer the mixture to an ice-cream maker, and freeze according to the manufacturer's instructions.

Nectarine Plum Cobbler

MAKES 4 SERVINGS

This raw version of a cobbler has a sweet, saucy fruit layer topped with crunchy nuts. While other fruits can easily be substituted for the nectarines, make sure you make the sauce from plums to create the right texture. Try this dessert with a scoop of Maple Walnut Ice Cream (see following recipe) for a special treat.

6 RIPE NECTARINES, PITTED AND SLICED INTO THIN WEDGES

6 RIPE RED OR BLACK PLUMS, PEELED, PITTED, AND CHOPPED

JUICE OF ½ LEMON

SEEDS FROM 1 VANILLA BEAN, SCRAPED

1 CUP ALMONDS, SOAKED IN WATER, FOR 8-12 HOURS,
    RINSED, AND DRAINED

1 CUP CASHEWS, SOAKED IN WATER, FOR 2-4 HOURS,
    RINSED, AND DRAINED

6-8 LARGE DATES, PITTED AND CHOPPED

½ TEASPOON GROUND NUTMEG

½ TEASPOON GROUND CINNAMON

DASH OF SEA SALT

1. Arrange the sliced nectarines in the bottom of a baking dish; set aside.

2. Place the plums, lemon juice, and vanilla seeds in a blender, and process until smooth. Pour over the nectarines.

3. Place the rest of the ingredients in a food processor, and pulse until the mixture resembles crumbs.

4. Spoon the crumble over the fruit and chill until served.

Maple Walnut Ice Cream

MAKES 6 CUPS

This simple two-ingredient recipe takes only a few hours to put together once the nuts have soaked. Don't cheat on the soaking time, or the texture of this ice cream will be grainy rather than smooth. If you like a bit of texture, add about half a cup of chopped walnuts to the ice cream while it is freezing.

6 CUPS WALNUTS SOAKED IN WATER FOR 10 HOURS, RINSED,
    AND DRAINED, RESERVING 1½ CUPS LIQUID
1½ CUPS PURE MAPLE SYRUP

1. Place the walnuts, reserved liquid, and maple syrup in a blender, and process until smooth.

2. Pour the mixture through a sieve, and then transfer the strained mixture to an ice-cream maker.

3. Freeze according to the manufacturer's instructions.

Chocolate Cashew Truffles

These decadent chocolate morsels are raw and delicious. Dust your hands in a little cocoa when rolling these truffles to keep the "ganache" from sticking. This is quite a messy recipe but completely worth the cleanup! You can also roll these truffles in freshly grated coconut or crushed nuts.

1½ CUPS CASHEW BUTTER

1½ CUPS PURE MAPLE SYRUP

1½ CUPS COCOA POWDER, PLUS MORE TO DUST TRUFFLES

SEEDS FROM 2 VANILLA BEANS, SCRAPED OUT

1. Place all the ingredients in a food processor, and process until thick and well blended.

2. Place the chocolate mixture in a bowl, and chill in the refrigerator until very firm.

3. Scrape out tablespoon-sized portions of the chocolate mixture, and roll each into a ball.

4. Roll the balls in cocoa powder, and store in the refrigerator in a sealed container.

French Vanilla Ice Cream

You will be hard-pressed to taste the difference between this raw ice cream and its custard-based counterpart. Both are creamy, flecked with vanilla seeds, and divine. You might choose to double this recipe if you have a large ice-cream maker, because it will become a staple dessert once you taste it.

3 CUPS FRESH CHOPPED COCONUT MEAT

3 CUPS UNSWEETENED COCONUT MILK

1½ CUPS PURE MAPLE SYRUP

1½ CUPS ALMOND MILK (SEE RECIPE IN CHAPTER 12)

⅓ CUP COCONUT OIL

SEEDS FROM 2 VANILLA BEANS, SCRAPED OUT

1. Place all the ingredients in a blender, and process until smooth and creamy.

2. Transfer the mixture to an ice-cream maker, and freeze according to the manufacturer's directions.

Luscious Lemon Bars

MAKES 16 SMALL SQUARES

These sweetly tart lemon bars are the perfect choice to bring to a potluck or family event. High in vitamin C, lemons are used by many people to detoxify and treat infections. If you wish, you can substitute lime for the lemon as long as the quantities remain the same.

FOR THE BASE:

1 CUP OLD-FASHIONED ROLLED OATS

1 CUP UNSWEETENED SHREDDED COCONUT

1 CUP PITTED DATES

FOR THE LEMON LAYER:

1 LARGE BANANA, PEELED

JUICE OF 4 LEMONS

⅔ CUP MELTED COCONUT OIL

⅔ CUP UNSWEETENED SHREDDED COCONUT

½ CUP PURE MAPLE SYRUP

Make the base:

1. Place all the ingredients in a food processor, and pulse until the mixture sticks together.

2. Press into the bottom of an 8 × 8–inch baking pan, and place in the refrigerator.

Make the lemon layer:

1. Place all the ingredients in a blender, and process until smooth. Adjust the taste for sweetness.

2. Spread the lemon layer onto the chilled base, and place the pan back in the refrigerator.

3. Chill for at least 12 hours, and cut into 16 squares.

CHAPTER TWELVE

Sauces and Staples

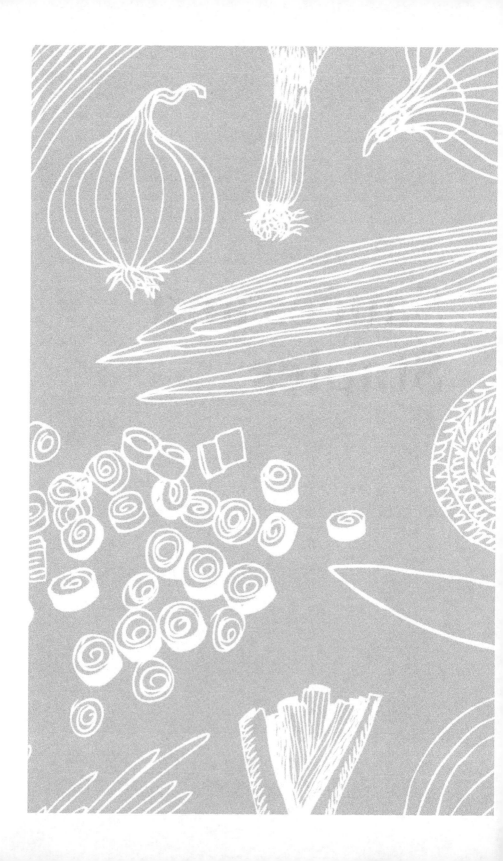

Raw Mayonnaise

MAKES 2 CUPS

This mayonnaise is so good you'll be tempted to eat it with a spoon. Slightly citrusy, light, fluffy, and very rich, it can be used as a spread, dip, or binding agent. If you wish, you can substitute macadamia nuts for the cashews, but that can be quite expensive.

2 CUPS CASHEWS, SOAKED IN WATER FOR 4-6 HOURS,
    RINSED, AND DRAINED
6 DATES, PITTED, SOAKED IN WATER FOR ABOUT
    10 MINUTES, AND DRAINED
½ CUP FRESH LEMON JUICE
½ CUP WATER
1 TABLESPOON ONION POWDER
1 TEASPOON GARLIC POWDER
½ CUP EXTRA-VIRGIN OLIVE OIL
1 TEASPOON SEA SALT, OR TO TASTE

1. Place all ingredients except the olive oil and sea salt in a blender, and puree until smooth, scraping down the sides.

2. Add the olive oil in a slow, steady stream until the mayonnaise emulsifies.

3. Season to taste with the sea salt.

Raspberry Vanilla Butter

MAKES 4 CUPS

While this spread can be made with other fruit, such as peaches, strawberries, and blueberries, raspberries tint the "butter" a luscious pink that is lovely spread on apples and raw pancakes. This recipe hardens up when stored in the refrigerator, so bring it to room temperature again before using it.

5 CUPS UNSWEETENED SHREDDED COCONUT

3 CUPS RASPBERRIES

3 TABLESPOONS AGAVE NECTAR

1 TABLESPOON FRESH LEMON JUICE

3 TEASPOONS PURE VANILLA EXTRACT

SEA SALT, TO TASTE

1. Place the coconut in a food processor, and blend until it has a butterlike consistency, about 10–15 minutes.

2. Add the remaining ingredients, and process until smooth, scraping down the sides.

3. Pass the vanilla butter through a very fine sieve, using the back of a spoon to remove the raspberry seeds.

4. Add more agave nectar, as needed.

5. Store in the refrigerator for up to 1 week. Let the spread come to room temperature before using.

Mango Chutney

Most traditional chutneys are cooked slowly and then served with roasted meats and patés. This raw version has the same complex, slightly hot spicing and chunky texture without the cooking and cooling. Use this chutney as a dip, or serve it alongside many raw stews or soups.

4 MEDIUM RIPE MANGOES, PEELED AND PITTED, DIVIDED
2 TABLESPOONS FINELY CHOPPED RED ONION
½ RED BELL PEPPER, FINELY CHOPPED
2 TABLESPOONS FRESH CHOPPED CILANTRO
1 TABLESPOON FRESH LEMON JUICE
1 TEASPOON MINCED FRESH GINGER
1 TEASPOON APPLE CIDER VINEGAR
½ TEASPOON GROUND CUMIN
SEA SALT, TO TASTE

1. Finely chop 3 mangos, and place them in a medium bowl.

2. Add the red onion and bell pepper, and stir to combine.

3. Place all the remaining ingredients except the sea salt in a blender, and pulse until smooth.

4. Add the blended ingredients to the mango mixture and toss to combine.

5. Season with the sea salt to taste.

6. Serve with chips or as a dip with vegetables.

Cucumber Coriander Dip

MAKES 4 CUPS

Coriander adds a lemony, almost currylike taste to dishes. Its flavor combines perfectly with cool cucumber and creamy cashew. Great with vegetables, this dip can be used to tone down the heat of raw chili or spicy soups.

MEAT OF 1 SMALL COCONUT

1 CUP CASHEWS, SOAKED IN WATER OVERNIGHT, RINSED,
　　AND DRAINED

⅓ CUP WATER

JUICE OF ½ LARGE LEMON

1 TEASPOON MINCED GARLIC

½ ENGLISH CUCUMBER, DICED

1 TEASPOON GROUND CORIANDER

½ TEASPOON GROUND CUMIN

1 TABLESPOON FRESH CHOPPED PARSLEY

SEA SALT AND FRESHLY GROUND BLACK PEPPER, TO TASTE

1. Process the coconut, cashews, water, lemon juice, and garlic in a blender until smooth.

2. Transfer the mixture to a bowl, and stir in the remaining ingredients.

3. Serve with vegetable chips or raw crackers.

Simple Almond Cheese

MAKES ABOUT 2 CUPS

Tasty and versatile, this almond cheese will become a staple in your repertoire. Experiment with other nuts to create different variations of the cheese. You can also use fresh herbs, spices, and even dried fruit to make one-of-a-kind cheeses for different occasions.

1½ CUPS ALMONDS, SOAKED IN WATER FOR 12 HOURS,
    RINSED, DRAINED, AND SKINS RUBBED OFF
1 CUP WATER
4 TABLESPOONS FRESH LEMON JUICE
5 TEASPOONS EXTRA-VIRGIN OLIVE OIL
1 HEAPING TEASPOON MINCED GARLIC
DASH OF SEA SALT

1. Place all the ingredients in a food processor, and process until smooth, scraping down the sides.

2. Transfer the almond mixture to a strainer lined with cheesecloth. Cover the top of the mixture with cheesecloth.

3. Set a light weight on top of the mixture, and place the strainer over another bowl to catch the liquid.

4. Place in the refrigerator overnight so the cheese can set up firm.

5. If you like softer cheese, use it straight from the refrigerator. For firmer cheese, place in a dehydrator for about 5 hours at 115 degrees F.

6. Store the cheese in the refrigerator for up to 5 days.

Cashew Sun-Dried Tomato Spread

MAKES ABOUT 2 CUPS

Sun-dried tomatoes pack a substantial flavor punch, and in this recipe they create an intense dip that can be used as a spread on many sandwiches and even tossed with vegetable noodles for a main course. You can double this recipe and store the extra in the refrigerator for up to a week.

1 CUP CASHEWS, SOAKED IN WATER FOR 10–12 HOURS,
    RINSED, AND DRAINED
¾ CUP SUN-DRIED TOMATOES, SOAKED IN WATER
    TO SOFTEN, DRAINED, AND CHOPPED
3 TABLESPOONS FRESH LEMON JUICE
2 TABLESPOONS DRIED BASIL OR DRIED OREGANO
SEA SALT AND FRESHLY GROUND
    BLACK PEPPER, TO TASTE

1. Place the cashews in a food processor, and pulse until they resemble ricotta cheese.

2. Transfer the processed nuts to a bowl, and add the remaining ingredients.

3. Chill in the refrigerator and use as a dip or as a spread.

Egg Salad

MAKES 3 CUPS

The success of this recipe depends on soaking the cashews for at least six hours, or the finished texture will be grainy rather than creamy. The turmeric gives a yellow hue to this mock egg salad, so add it little by little until you obtain the desired shade. As with real egg salad, feel free to add extras such as carrots or onions.

2 CUPS CASHEWS, SOAKED IN WATER FOR 6 HOURS,
    RINSED, AND DRAINED
1 CUP WATER
JUICE AND ZEST OF 2 LARGE LEMONS
1 TEASPOON MINCED GARLIC
1 TEASPOON SEA SALT
1 TEASPOON GROUND TURMERIC, OR AS NEEDED
2 STALKS CELERY, FINELY CHOPPED
2 SCALLIONS, CHOPPED
FRESHLY GROUND BLACK PEPPER, TO TASTE
PAPRIKA, FOR GARNISH
LETTUCE CUPS OR RAW BREAD, FOR SERVING

1. Place the cashews, water, lemon juice, lemon zest, garlic, sea salt, and turmeric in a blender, and pulse until smooth.

2. Transfer the mixture to a medium bowl, and add the celery and scallions; stir to combine.

3. Season with the black pepper to taste and top with paprika.

4. Serve in lettuce cups or on raw bread.

Raw Tortilla

MAKES 4 TORTILLAS

You wouldn't think zucchini could create a tortilla that is quite close to its wheat-based cousin, but it does. The trick to these wraps is exact timing in the dehydrator. Too little time will create wet wraps that rip, and too much time will make them crispy and prone to cracking. Follow the directions carefully to ensure that your tortillas come out perfectly.

6 CUPS PEELED GREEN ZUCCHINI

¼ CUP EXTRA-VIRGIN OLIVE OIL

2 TABLESPOONS FRESH LEMON JUICE

1 TABLESPOON GROUND CORIANDER

1 TEASPOON SEA SALT

PINCH OF CAYENNE PEPPER

1 CUP GROUND FLAXSEED

1. Place all the ingredients except the flaxseed in a blender, and pulse until smooth.

2. Add the flaxseed to the blender, and pulse again until the mixture is smooth.

3. Pour the mixture evenly between 4 dehydrator sheets with nonstick pads on them, forming a rough circle on each sheet.

4. Dehydrate the tortillas at 105 degrees F for 7–8 hours, or until the tortillas peel off the sheets easily.

5. Remove the tortillas from the nonstick pads, and place them directly on the dehydrator sheets. Put them back in the dehydrator for about 45 minutes, until they are dry to the touch but still pliable.

6. Wrap the tortillas around your favorite fillings and serve.

Simple Almond Butter

MAKES 2 CUPS

You can use pretty much any type of nut or seed to create different types of butters with this recipe. Processing the almonds will take ten to twenty minutes, depending on your food processor. To get a uniform texture, stop the machine periodically to scrape down the sides.

4 CUPS ALMONDS

1. Place the almonds in a food processor, and process until the butter is smooth and shiny.

Almond Tart Base

MAKES 10–12 TART SHELLS

This almost buttery tart base has a tender crispness that makes it perfect for many fillings. For a more finished-looking tart, you can also press this mixture into little tart pans before the dehydration process. Simply pop them out when they feel crisp on top, and place them back in the dehydrator upside down for another hour.

1½ CUPS ALMOND FLOUR
¾ CUP GROUND FLAXSEED
½ CUP ALMOND BUTTER
½ CUP FINELY GRATED CARROT, LIQUID SQUEEZED OUT
¼ CUP WATER
PINCH OF SEA SALT
FRESH FRUIT, FOR SERVING

1. Place all the ingredients except the fresh fruit in a food processor, and pulse until they come together like dough.

2. Transfer the dough to a sheet of plastic wrap, and wrap it tightly.

3. Place the dough in the refrigerator for about 1 hour to make it easier to handle.

4. Remove the dough from the refrigerator and flatten it into a round between two nonstick sheets. Roll out to a ⅛-inch thickness.

5. Using a cookie cutter or a drinking glass, cut the dough into rounds about 3 inches in diameter.

6. Use your fingers to make a raised rim around the edge of the tarts.

7. Place the tart shells on a dehydrator sheet, and dehydrate for about 2 hours at 105 degrees F until dry.

8. Refrigerate until needed, and serve filled with fresh fruit.

Raw Sour Cream

MAKES 4 CUPS

In a blind taste test you wouldn't be able to tell this raw sour cream apart from the real deal. Make sure you soak your nuts for the recommended time. You want the texture of this sour cream to be smooth rather than grainy.

3 CUPS FRESH CHOPPED COCONUT MEAT

1½ CUPS CASHEWS, SOAKED IN WATER FOR 10–12 HOURS, RINSED, AND DRAINED

⅓ CUP FRESH LEMON JUICE

⅓ CUP EXTRA-VIRGIN OLIVE OIL

3 TEASPOONS PUREED DATES

½ TEASPOON SEA SALT, OR TO TASTE

1½ CUPS WATER, OR AS NEEDED

1. Process all the ingredients except the water in a blender until smooth.

2. Transfer the mixture to a bowl, and stir in the water until you reach the desired thickness.

3. Store the sour cream in a covered container in the refrigerator for up to 1 week.

Almond Milk

You will be creating two raw food staples when you make this recipe—the strained almond milk and the leftover almond pulp that can be used as flour. Try using other nuts for variations that can be used in recipes or enjoyed as a refreshing and nutritious beverage.

4 CUPS ALMONDS
8 CUPS WATER

1. Place the almonds in an uncovered bowl and cover with approximately 1 inch of water. Let stand overnight, and up to 2 days. (The longer the almonds soak, the creamier the almond milk.)

2. Drain the almonds and rinse thoroughly in cool running water.

3. Place the almonds and water in a blender, and process until almonds are a fine meal and water is opaque.

4. Line a large bowl with two layers of fine cheesecloth, letting it drape over the edges.

5. Pour the almond mixture into the bowl, and bring the corners of the cloth up, creating a bag.

6. Squeeze out as much liquid as possible, twisting the bag.

7. Transfer the pulp to a lidded container to use as almond flour.

8. Store the almond milk in the refrigerator for up to 4 days.

Tangy Sauerkraut

Sauerkraut has been made in bowls and jars for centuries in many different countries. The fermentation method is called "lacto-fermentation," which means it does not use heat. It is important to let the cabbage ferment long enough to get the full tangy taste. Feel free to use red cabbage in place of green, or a combination of the two.

2 HEADS GREEN CABBAGE, FINELY SHREDDED
　　(SAVE ABOUT 8 LARGE OUTER LEAVES)
¼ CUP SEA SALT

1. Place the shredded cabbage in a very large bowl, layering it with the salt.

2. Press down on the top of the cabbage until liquid starts to drain a little.

3. Cover the top of the cabbage with the reserved leaves, and cover those with plastic wrap.

4. Place 2 or 3 weights on top of the plastic, and set the bowl on the counter. After about 24 hours, check to see if the liquid rises above the level of the cabbage. If it is too low, add a little salt water (1 teaspoon of salt in 1 cup water).

5. Let the sauerkraut sit for 3–6 days until it is well fermented and smells tangy. You might see a layer of gray mold on the reserved leaves. Simply remove the leaves before packing the sauerkraut into sterilized liter jars.

6. Store in the refrigerator. Sauerkraut will keep for up to 2 months in a covered container.

Creamy Vanilla Yogurt

MAKES 5 CUPS

Yogurt is one of those food items that most new raw foodists miss intensely, so this recipe is a wonderful discovery. Probiotic powder can be purchased in many grocery or specialty food stores and is usually found in capsules. Simply open up the capsule and add it to the other ingredients. Make sure you taste the yogurt while it sits. It becomes tangier with time.

4 CUPS FRESH COCONUT MEAT
1½ CUPS COCONUT WATER
SEEDS FROM 1 VANILLA BEAN, SCRAPED OUT
¼ CUP AGAVE NECTAR
1 TEASPOON PROBIOTIC POWDER

1. Place the coconut meat and coconut water in a food processor, and process until smooth and creamy.

2. Add the vanilla seeds and agave nectar, and process until well blended.

3. Add the probiotic powder, and process until well incorporated.

4. Transfer the yogurt to a container, and store sealed in the refrigerator until it tastes like yogurt, about 16–18 hours.

5. Store in the refrigerator. Yogurt will keep for 5–6 days.

Indonesian Peanut Sauce

MAKES 3 CUPS

This spicy, sweet sauce has a complex heat that can sneak up on you. Use it to enhance other raw food dishes, or serve it spooned over parsnip or cauliflower rice. It also makes a great dip for vegetables.

2 CUPS RAW PEANUT BUTTER

1 CUP RAW HONEY

½ CUP FRESH LEMON JUICE

½ CUP TOASTED SESAME OIL

¼ CUP TAHINI

2 TABLESPOONS NAMA SHOYU

1 TABLESPOON RED CHILI FLAKES, OR TO TASTE

WATER, TO THIN THE SAUCE

1. Place all the ingredients except the chili flakes and water in a blender, and blend until smooth.

2. Add the chili flakes to taste, and thin the mixture with water if the sauce is too thick.

3. Store the sauce in a sealed container in the refrigerator for up to 1 week.

CHAPTER THIRTEEN

Snacks and Kid-Friendly Recipes

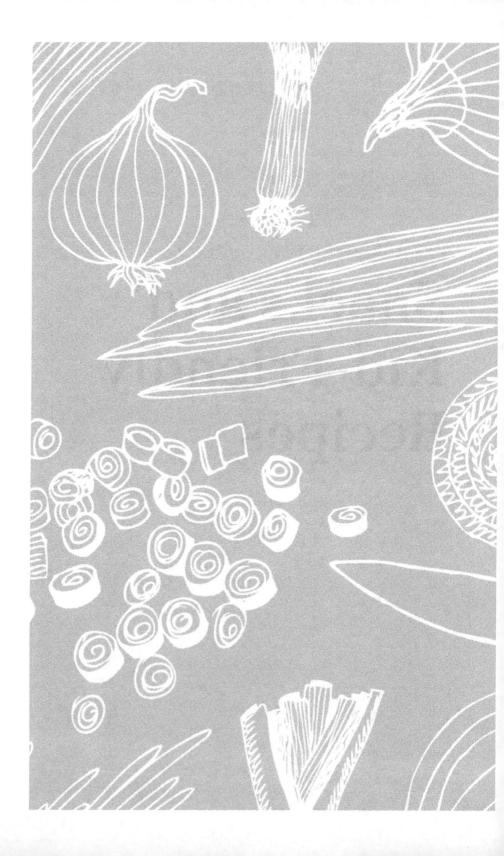

Candied Almonds

MAKES 4 CUPS

These tempting treats beg to be tucked into tidy little packages and given as gifts to the special people in your life. Sweet and crunchy, they can be dusted with cinnamon or nutmeg, if desired. You can also try this recipe with pecans or walnuts.

4 CUPS ALMONDS, SOAKED IN WATER FOR 6 HOURS,
　　RINSED, DRAINED, AND PATTED DRY
½ CUP PURE MAPLE SYRUP
¼ CUP ORANGE ZEST

1. In a medium bowl, toss together the almonds and maple syrup until the nuts are well coated.

2. Spread the almonds on several nonstick sheets, and dehydrate for 6–8 hours at 105 degrees F.

3. Turn the almonds over and dehydrate for 18–20 hours until very crisp, adding the orange zest halfway through the time.

4. Transfer the almonds to a sealed container.

Tempting Caramel Apples

MAKES 8 CARAMEL APPLES

Halloween. Brisk fall days. Children's parties and special events. That is what these amazing toffee-wrapped apples evoke, even though they can be made year-round. Applying the caramel needs a little supervision to ensure that the thickness is just right. If you don't get perfectly covered apples, don't worry. Simply pour the caramel into a bowl and dip apple wedges into it instead.

2 CUPS CASHEWS, SOAKED IN WATER FOR 4 HOURS,
    RINSED, AND DRAINED
⅔ CUP PURE MAPLE SYRUP
½ CUP WATER
¼ CUP COCONUT OIL
2 TABLESPOONS PURE VANILLA EXTRACT
DASH OF SEA SALT
8 FIRM APPLES, STEMS REMOVED
8 WOODEN CRAFT STICKS
2 CUPS FINELY CHOPPED ALMONDS, DEHYDRATED UNTIL DRY

1. Put all the ingredients except the apples, craft sticks, and almonds in a blender, and process until smooth, almost creamy.

2. Transfer the mixture to a deep bowl, and store it in the refrigerator until thick.

3. Press the craft sticks firmly into the bottom of the apples. Thoroughly dry the apples with paper towels.

4. Dip the apples into the caramel until completely covered, letting any excess drip off; then roll the apples in the chopped almonds.

5. Place the apples on wax paper, and chill in the refrigerator until firm.

Chia Chocolate Pudding Bowl

Don't make this recipe in a small bowl. Chia seeds swell up to nine times their volume as they sit in liquid. The chocolaty taste in this pudding is not intense. If you want a stronger chocolate kick, simply add more cocoa and sweetener.

9 TABLESPOONS CHIA SEEDS
4½ CUPS ALMOND MILK (SEE RECIPE IN CHAPTER 12)
3 TEASPOONS AGAVE NECTAR
3 TABLESPOONS COCOA POWDER
SEEDS FROM 2 VANILLA BEANS, SCRAPED OUT

1. In a medium bowl combine all the ingredients until well blended.

2. Place the bowl in the refrigerator for about 30 minutes until the pudding is thick.

Watermelon-Strawberry Ice Pops

MAKES 6 ICE POPS

Ice pops scream summer. Who hasn't sat on a dock swinging their legs and holding a dripping sticky Popsicle in the sun as a kid? If not, then make these refreshing pink treats and find the nearest dock. You can use almost any fruit, but the combination of watermelon and ripe strawberries is exceptional.

1 CUP CUBED SEEDLESS WATERMELON
2 CUPS SLICED STRAWBERRIES

1. Place the fruit in a blender and process until smooth.

2. Pour the liquid through a sieve to remove the strawberry and watermelon seeds.

3. Pour the liquid into 6 ice-pop molds and freeze.

Spiced Eggplant Chips

Some people don't care for eggplant because its texture can be porous and it can sometimes taste bitter. These chips are a nice surprise in their crispiness and spicy flavor. The initial stage in the dehydrator uses a higher temperature than what is usually recommended for raw food, but since the eggplant never reaches that temperature, it is okay. You can use different spices and herbs on these chips for tasty variations.

3 EGGPLANTS, PEELED AND THINLY SLICED
⅓ CUP EXTRA-VIRGIN OLIVE OIL
⅔ CUP WATER
3 TEASPOONS AGAVE NECTAR
1 TABLESPOON SMOKED PAPRIKA
½ TEASPOON GROUND CHIPOTLE

1. Place the sliced eggplant in a large bowl.

2. In a small bowl, stir together the rest of the ingredients until well combined.

3. Add the wet ingredients to the sliced eggplant, and stir to combine.

4. Place the bowl in the refrigerator overnight to marinate.

5. Place the slices in a dehydrator, and dehydrate for about 1 hour at 145 degrees F.

6. Reduce the heat to 115 degrees F and dehydrate for about 8 hours, or until the chips are crispy.

7. Serve with or without a dip.

Cocoa Pecan Fudge

Fudge is a guilty pleasure. This recipe creates slightly nutty, intensely chocolate nuggets of simple decadence. Omit the pecans if you want a pure chocolate experience. To get neat squares, don't cut the fudge until it is firm, no matter how much you want to try them.

1½ CUPS ALMOND BUTTER, AT ROOM TEMPERATURE
¾ CUP COCOA POWDER
⅓ CUP AGAVE NECTAR
½ CUP CHOPPED PECANS

1. Line a 9 × 13–inch baking dish with parchment paper and set aside.

2. In a large bowl, stir together the almond butter, cocoa powder, and agave nectar until well blended.

3. Add the chopped pecans and stir to combine.

4. Spread the fudge into the prepared baking dish, and place in the refrigerator for at least 3 hours until firm.

5. Cut the fudge into squares, and store in the freezer or refrigerator in a sealed container.

Garden Roll-ups

MAKES 4 (2-ROLL) SERVINGS

Wraps are popular because they are convenient finger food. While this version takes a bit of work to make, it is well worth the effort. The trick to picking up these wraps is making sure you squeeze out the moisture from your vegetables, or the wrap will be too soggy to work with or eat easily. Try these wraps with a little peanut dipping sauce or a dab of raw sour cream.

1 CUP SHREDDED RED CABBAGE

1 CUP SHREDDED BABY SPINACH

2 LARGE CARROTS, PEELED AND GRATED

1 RED BELL PEPPER, SEEDED AND SLICED INTO THIN STRIPS

3 SCALLIONS, GREEN AND WHITE PARTS THINLY SLICED

1 TABLESPOON FRESH LEMON JUICE

SEA SALT AND FRESHLY GROUND BLACK PEPPER, TO TASTE

2 LARGE CUCUMBERS, SKIN LEFT ON AND SLICED INTO THIN RIBBONS

¼ CUP HERB PESTO

2 CUPS ALFALFA SPOUTS

1. In a large bowl, toss together the cabbage, spinach, carrots, bell pepper, scallions, and lemon juice until well combined.

2. Season to taste with the sea salt and black pepper.

3. Place the cucumber slices on paper towels to drain.

4. Place 4 drained cucumber slices on a flat work surface, overlapping them slightly along the entire length.

5. Spread about 1 teaspoon of the herb pesto on the cucumber slices.

6. Place 1 spoonful of vegetables and a small handful of the alfalfa sprouts on one end of the slices.

7. Roll the cucumber slices around the vegetables, and place the rolls on a plate seam side down.

Rich Chocolate Shake

Remember old-fashioned chocolate malted shakes? Then you will be delighted with this raw version. It is so thick you might find yourself using a spoon instead of straw. Don't omit the little bit of salt in the recipe. It actually enhances the sweetness and chocolaty taste.

½ CUP CASHEWS, SOAKED IN WATER FOR 5 HOURS,
 RINSED, AND DRAINED
½ CUP ALMOND MILK (SEE RECIPE IN CHAPTER 12)
SEEDS FROM 1 VANILLA BEAN, SCRAPED OUT
¼ CUP COCOA POWDER
2 TABLESPOONS UNSWEETENED FLAKED COCONUT
2 TABLESPOONS RAW HONEY
½ RIPE AVOCADO, PEELED AND PITTED
1 CUP ICE CUBES

1. Place all the ingredients except the ice cubes in a blender, and process until smooth.

2. Add the ice cubes, and blend until thick and smooth.

Almond Praline

MAKES 6 SERVINGS

Praline is a snack, topping, and tasty gift idea rolled into one sweet package. For a variation, try making this recipe with pecans, walnuts, or pistachios. If you live in a humid climate, you might find the finished product a little sticky. If so, store the praline between layers of waxed paper instead of stacking the pieces directly on top of each other.

3 CUPS CHOPPED ALMONDS, SOAKED IN WATER FOR
    8 HOURS, RINSED, AND DRAINED
⅔ CUP PURE MAPLE SYRUP
1 TEASPOON GROUND CINNAMON
½ TEASPOON FRESHLY GRATED NUTMEG
PINCH OF SEA SALT

1. Combine all the ingredients in a large bowl until well mixed.

2. Transfer the almond mixture to a nonstick drying sheet, and spread it out evenly.

3. Dehydrate for 8–10 hours at 105 degrees F until crisp.

4. Remove and break the praline into pieces.

5. Store in an airtight container.

Sweet Potato Chips

MAKES 4 SERVINGS

Chips are the snack of choice for kids and adults alike, and these salty-sweet, golden beauties are healthful and delicious. To create perfectly crisp chips, make sure each sweet potato slice is evenly coated with olive oil and that the slices are not overlapping on the dehydrator screen.

3 LARGE SWEET POTATOES, SKIN LEFT ON AND THINLY SLICED
    (WITH A MANDOLINE, IF POSSIBLE)
¼ CUP EXTRA-VIRGIN OLIVE OIL
SEA SALT AND FRESHLY GROUND BLACK PEPPER, TO TASTE
DASH OF GROUND CINNAMON OR CAYENNE PEPPER

1. Toss the sweet potato slices with olive oil and seasonings until they are well coated.

2. Spread the slices on several mesh dehydrator trays, making sure they don't overlap.

3. Dehydrate the chips for 10–12 hours at 115 degrees F.

Glossary

agave nectar A liquid sweetener taken from the agave plant, with a low glycemic load. It is a great substitute for sugar.

cacao nibs The part of the cocoa bean that is edible after the bean is processed.

cocoa powder The powder produced after cacao nibs are ground, the cocoa butter is extracted from the nibs, and the leftover brown paste is dried and ground again.

coconut butter The meat and oil of the coconut pureed into a smooth butter.

coconut oil The oil that is extracted from the meat of the coconut.

coconut water The clear, nutrient-packed water found in young coconuts.

Ezekiel wrap A sprouted-grain wrap that is appropriate for a raw diet.

flaxseed The seeds from the flax plant. Flaxseed is used extensively in raw recipes, are very high in many nutrients, and can also be sprouted or ground.

green smoothie A blended beverage made from green leafy vegetables and combined with fruit.

miso A traditional Japanese product made by fermenting rice, barley, and/or soybeans with salt and koji (a fungus). Miso is widely used to enhance many recipes and finished dishes.

nama shoyu A Japanese unpasteurized soy sauce, which is considered a good choice for a raw diet.

nutritional yeast A nutritional supplement used as a protein source and as a substitute for cheese in vegan and raw cuisine.

probiotics Live bacteria that are thought to positively impact the digestive system.

sea salt A natural and unrefined salt that is considered to be more healthful than processed salts.

tahini A paste made from ground sesame seeds. Tahini is used in many Middle Eastern dishes.

vanilla beans The seed pods of a vanilla vine.

vegan A diet that does not include any animal products, eggs, dairy products, or other animal-derived substances, such as gelatin.

Daily Nutrients Charts

	RECOMMENDED DAILY NUTRIENTS							
	FEMALES							
	11 to 14	15 to 18	19 to 24	20 to 50	51 +	Pregnant	Lactating months 1 to 12	Lactating months 13 to 16
Energy (kcal)	2200	2200	2200	2200	1900	Plus 300	Plus 500	2200
Carbs (grams)	300	300	300	300	300	300	Plus 500	300
Sugar (grams)	100	100	100	100	100	100	100	100
Proteins (grams)	46	44	46	50	50	60	65	62
Calcium (mg)	1200	1200	1200	800	800	1200	1200	1200
B1 (mg)	1.1	1.1	1.1	1.1	1	1.5	1.6	1.6
B2 (mg)	1.3	1.3	1.3	1.3	1.2	1.6	1.8	1.7
B3 (mg)	15	15	15	15	13	17	20	20
B6 (mg)	2	2	2	2	2	2.2	2.6	2.6
B12 (mg)	2	2	2	2	2	2.2	2.6	2.6
Vitamin C (mg)	50	60	60	60	60	70	95	90
Vitamin D (mg)	10	10	10	5	5	10	10	10
Vitamin E (mcg)	8	8	8	8	8	10	12	11
Vitamin K (mcg)	45	55	60	65	65	65	65	65
Phosphorus (mg)	1200	1200	1200	800	800	1200	1200	1200
Magnesium (mg)	280	300	280	280	280	320	355	340
Iron (mg)	15	15	15	15	10	30	15	15
Zinc (mcg)	12	12	12	12	12	15	19	16
Selenium (mcg)	45	50	55	55	55	65	75	75
Iodine (mcg)	150	150	150	150	150	175	200	200

RECOMMENDED DAILY NUTRIENTS							
	CHILDREN		MALES				
	4 to 6	7 to 10	11 to 14	15 to 18	19 to 24	25 to 50	51 +
Energy (kcal)	1800	2400	2500	3000	2900	2900	2300
Carbs (grams)	130	150	300	300	300	300	300
Sugar (grams)	100	100	100	100	100	100	100
Proteins (grams)	30	36	45	59	58	63	63
Calcium (mg)	800	800	1200	1200	1200	800	800
B1 (mg)	0.9	1	1.3	1.5	1.5	1.5	1.2
B2 (mg)	1.1	1.2	1.5	1.8	1.7	1.7	1.4
B3 (mg)	12	13	17	20	19	19	15
B6 (mg)	1.1	1.2	1.7	2	2	2	2
B12 (mg)	1.5	2	2	2	2	2	2
Vitamin C (mg)	45	45	50	60	60	60	60
Vitamin D (mg)	5	5	10	10	10	5	5
Vitamin E (mcg)	7	7	10	10	10	10	10
Vitamin K (mcg)	20	30	45	65	70	80	80
Phosphorus (mg)	500	800	1200	1200	1200	800	800
Magnesium (mg)	130	150	270	400	350	350	350
Iron (mg)	10	10	12	12	10	10	10
Zinc (mcg)	10	10	15	15	15	15	15
Selenium (mcg)	20	30	40	50	70	70	70
Iodine (mcg)	90	100	150	150	150	150	150

Index

Lightning Source UK Ltd.
Milton Keynes UK
UKHW020245181221
395826UK00009B/549